FINANCE
—— *and* ——
BUDGETING
Made Simple
Essential Skills for Nurses

KT Waxman, DNP, MBA, RN, CNL, CENP, CHSE

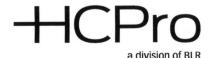

a division of BLR

Finance and Budgeting Made Simple: Essential Skills for Nurses is published by HCPro, a division of BLR.

Download the additional materials of this book at *www.hcpro.com/downloads/12427*

ISBN: 978-1-55645-520-9

HCPro provides information resources for the healthcare industry.

HCPro is not affiliated in any way with The Joint Commission, which owns the JCAHO and Joint Commission trademarks.

KT Waxman, DNP, MBA, RN, CNL, CENP, CHSE, Author
Rebecca Hendren, Editor
Erin Callahan, Senior Director, Product
Elizabeth Petersen, Vice President
Matt Sharpe, Production Supervisor
Vincent Skyers, Design Services Director
Vicki McMahan, Sr. Graphic Designer
Jason Gregory, Layout/Graphic Design
Tyson Davis, Cover Designer

Advice given is general. Readers should consult professional counsel for specific legal, ethical, or clinical questions.

Arrangements can be made for quantity discounts. For more information, contact:

HCPro
100 Winners Circle
Suite 300
Brentwood, TN 37027
Telephone: 800-650-6787 or 781-639-1872
Fax: 800-785-9212 Email: *customerservice@hcpro.com*

Visit HCPro online at *www.hcpro.com* and *www.hcmarketplace.com*

Contents

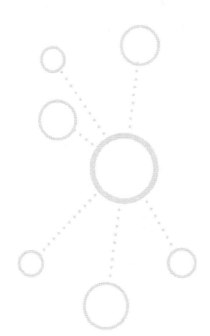

About the Author

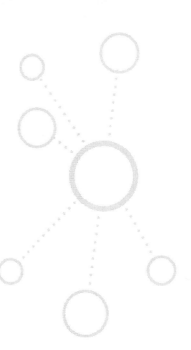

KT Waxman, DNP, MBA, RN, CNL, CENP, CHSE, is a nurse leader with more than 30 years of experience in healthcare and corporate settings. She is a tenured assistant professor at the University of San Francisco School of Nursing and Health Professions. She is chair of the Healthcare Leadership and Innovations department, which includes the Doctor of Nursing Practice (DNP) and Masters in Healthcare Simulation programs. As the director of the Department of Defense grant funded simulation research study, she completed a study on medication error recognition and simulation modalities.

Dr. Waxman is also director of the California Simulation Alliance (CSA) at the California Institute for Nursing & Health Care (CINHC). An internationally known speaker and author, she is past president of the Association of California Nurse Leaders (ACNL) and currently serves as treasurer of the American Organization of Nurse Executives (AONE), a 9,000-member association. She served as cochair of the International Meeting on Simulation in Healthcare for the Society for Simulation in Healthcare (SSH) in 2012 and is currently serving on the oversight committee.

Dr. Waxman's work has been published extensively and can be found in journals such as *Simulation in Healthcare, Clinical Simulation for Nursing, Journal of Nursing Education, Nurse Leader, Creative Nursing,* and *MedSim.* She is a chapter author for three simulation textbooks. She is the author of the books *A Practical Guide to Finance and Budgeting: Skills for Nurse Managers,* published by HCPro, and *Financial and Business Management for the Doctor of Nursing Practice, published* by Springer in 2012.

Waxman received her DNP from the University of San Francisco, with an emphasis on health systems leadership and a concentration in clinical simulation. She holds national certifications as a Clinical Nurse Leader (CNL), a Nurse Executive (CENP), and a Healthcare Simulation Educator (CHSE).

About the Book

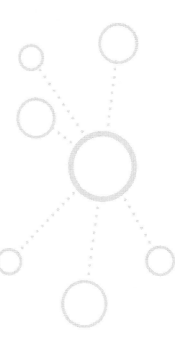

All the book's resources are available to download and customize for your practice, including bonus tools not featured in the book.

To access the resources, please visit: *www.hcpro.com/downloads/12427*

Continuing Education

Nursing contact hours

HCPro is accredited as a provider of continuing nursing education by the American Nurses Credentialing Center's Commission on Accreditation.

This educational activity for 2 nursing contact hours is provided by HCPro.

Nursing contact hours for this activity are valid from June 2015 until June 2018.

For complete information about credits available and instructions on how to take the continuing education exam, please visit the downloads page and see the Nursing Education Instructional Guide at *www.hcpro.com/downloads/12427.*

Disclosure statement

The planners, presenters/authors, and contributors of this CNE activity have disclosed no relevant financial relationships with any commercial companies pertaining to this activity.

Learning objectives

After reading this book, the participants should be able to:

- Read and understand healthcare financial statements

- Identify the flow of the revenue cycle in their facility

- Discuss the foreign language of finance

- Understand the nurse manager's role in operating a unit as a "business"

- Identify the components of a financial statement

- Explain the differences between a balance sheet, income statement and departmental operating report, and income and departmental expenditures

- Describe the process of budgeting for staff, supplies, equipment, and capital expenditures

- Identify the process to construct a budget

- Describe breakeven analysis

- Define controllable costs

- Explain how to manage variances in their budget

- Identify the components of a business case

- Understand return on investment (ROI)

- Articulate why building a business case is important to secure necessary resources

Leadership Dimensions and Processes

Learning Objectives

After reading this chapter, the learners will be able to:

- Read and understand healthcare financial statements
- Identify the flow of the revenue cycle in their facility
- Discuss the foreign language of finance
- Understand the nurse manager's role in operating a unit as a "business"

Today's Nurse Manager

There is no question that in today's healthcare environment the role of the nurse manager is very different than it was 25 years ago. Back then, nurse managers were referred to as head nurses and were responsible for leading their area or unit in a much different capacity than is expected today. Head nurses were primarily responsible for providing patient care and running the unit and were often considered working supervisors. Fast forward to the present, and the term head nurse is virtually extinct.

This is not to say that the duties of head nurses no longer exist; on the contrary, they have multiplied. Now you find those responsible for overseeing the same tasks as head nurses donning titles such as nurse managers, directors, coordinators, and service-line leaders, with each title dependent on the healthcare setting in which they work.

These leaders, regardless of their titles, are responsible for managing and guiding their units 24 hours a day, seven days a week. Nowadays, additional skills beyond the clinical base are necessary to do the job. This book will discuss and explain one of the necessary skills for the successful nurse manager: financial management.

Responsibilities

The authority and responsibilities of nurse managers differ from organization to organization. However, there are some core competencies that are required consistently. Interpersonal skills, resource management, time management, communication skills, and a clinical background are all part of the nurse manager's repertoire.

According to the American Organization of Nurse Executives (AONE), some of the essential competencies of nurse managers include the following:

The Science: Managing the business:

- Financial management

- Human resource management

- Performance improvement

- Foundational thinking skills

- Technology

- Strategic management

- Clinical practice knowledge

The Leader Within: Creating the leader in yourself:

- Personal and professional accountability

- Career planning

- Personal journey disciplines

- Optimizing the leader within

The Art: Leading the people

- Human resource leadership skills
- Relationship management and influencing behaviors
- Diversity
- Shared decision-making

Source: Nurse Manager Leadership Partnership Learning Domain Framework

Within the financial management competency, the objectives are as follows:

- Develop a practical annual budget for a unit or department that includes volume, revenue, personnel, supplies, and capital equipment
- Give weekly or monthly reports of budgetary variances to your supervisor and review end-of-year data with the finance department and the Chief Nursing Officer (CNO)
- Ensure proper, efficient operations, and monitor trends regarding staff, material, and supply usage
- Communicate fiscal management expectations and outcomes to your staff and other stakeholders
- Understand healthcare reform, value-based purchasing, and revenue cycle as it relates to your unit

Education and training

The majority of the nurse manager's education focuses on clinical nursing. Because you have picked up this book, it's safe to assume that you are just one of the many clinically proficient staff nurses who have been promoted to nurse manager without any formal or informal business or financial experience or training. This side of nurse managing likely causes the most strife and warrants the most education.

Whether you go out and get this training yourself or your hospital makes it available to you, learning the skills necessary to be a manager is vital to your career. To become a successful financial manager, you must know and learn tasks such as creating and presenting budgets, reading financial statements, and managing the financial aspects of the units.

Of course, this is not to say that you should forsake your clinical training. On the contrary, use it to your fullest advantage. As a nurse with business acumen and finance knowledge, you will carry a particularly important position, because you can inject your clinical knowledge into the budgeting process. By doing so, you help ensure that patients continue to get safe, quality care even when budget cuts must be made. Begin by learning what makes the financial hearts of hospitals and healthcare organizations tick.

This Is a Business

Now that you are a financial manager, the main point to remember is that hospitals and other healthcare organizations are businesses. And for businesses to be successful, they must make a profit on the goods or services they offer or sell.

Many hospitals are not-for-profit. Such organizations generally use earnings to construct new buildings, provide raises for staff, or buy new equipment. For-profit hospitals essentially spend their earnings on the same things; however, they have the additional expense of paying back shareholders.

As with every business, there are certain politics that dictate hospitals' operations. Therefore, you as a financial manager must understand the politics behind healthcare economics.

The Current Healthcare Environment

Healthcare reform has arrived. One of the focuses of the Affordable Care Act (ACA) is to insure more people. In 2006, more than 47 million people were uninsured. After the institution of the ACA, 41 million were uninsured, which is approximately 13% of the U.S. population. Other components of the ACA (which is 2,409 pages long!) are:

- Improving quality and efficiency
- Prevention of chronic disease and improving health
- Increasing the healthcare workforce
- Improving access to innovative therapies
- Community living assisted services and support
- Changing payment structure
- Revenue provisions
- Strengthening quality for all

The ACA has required the Centers for Medicare & Medicaid Services (CMS) to establish a shared savings program, bundled payment models, and value-based purchasing (VBP). These models and components of the ACA are important for nurse managers to understand, as controlling costs is key to reimbursement.

VBP is also known as pay for performance and is intended to realign hospital or healthcare organization financial incentives by rewarding them for achieving specific quality outcomes. On the flip side, they will be penalized for failing to do so.

The state of the economy plays a large role in increasing healthcare costs. During rough economic times, many consumers must make the harsh decision of whether to put food on the table or pay for healthcare. As you can imagine, many neglect their health until they are ill, entering the healthcare system through the emergency department, which increases costs significantly. Although the ACA will address some of these issues, many will still be uninsured, continue to have chronic disease, and use emergency departments, thus increasing costs.

Another major factor in increasing healthcare costs is the overall shortage of healthcare workers in the nation, particularly RNs. When hospitals have high RN vacancy rates, they must resort to alternatives, such as using costly contract/agency staff and offering incentive programs such as sign-on bonuses. They also use traveling nurses, who work on minimum 13-week assignments, to fill open slots within hospitals at a higher rate of pay. These actions are short-term solutions and significantly increase hospital expenditures.

Technology and Pharmaceuticals

The cost of technology plays a major role in the cost of healthcare, and there has been an explosion of available technology in the past 25 years. The more technology that is available, the more there is a need for specialists to run the technology. Hospitals, competing for the best physicians to come on staff to attract more patients, buy expensive technologies.

In the past, hospitals were paid by the various health insurers each time a procedure was performed with new equipment. Today, with healthcare reform, procedures are not reimbursed separately; rather, the hospital receives a flat-rate reimbursement.

Hospitals feel it is necessary to have the most current technology to attract patients and physicians, but it can be costly. In addition, with increased litigation in the industry, physicians are more apt to order pricey, high-tech tests to ensure that they have covered all bases to avoid a lawsuit. They essentially order tests for the benefit of the medical record, not for the patient.

The number of new medications developed in the pharmaceutical industry has skyrocketed over the past 25 years, thus increasing the cost of healthcare. As these drugs become available and are used by physicians, it adds to the costs of patient care. This is because the costs to develop, test, and approve new medications are high, and it can take years before a medication reaches the marketplace. When the medication is finally available to the public, manufacturers must charge enough to cover these costs and pay their stockholders, who expect to see a return on their investment. The price of drugs does not drop significantly until companies begin to sell generic versions.

Healthcare Spending

Understanding how the United States spends its money on healthcare and how it relates to the gross domestic product (GDP) is important. Figure 1.1 from the OECD from 2010 shows the national health expenditures compared to other countries. You can see in the chart that the United States spends almost twice as much as most countries, yet our outcomes are no better than theirs. In some cases, such as our life expectancy, our outcomes are unfavorable. The average U.S. life expectancy is 79.56 and we are ranked number 42 in the world.

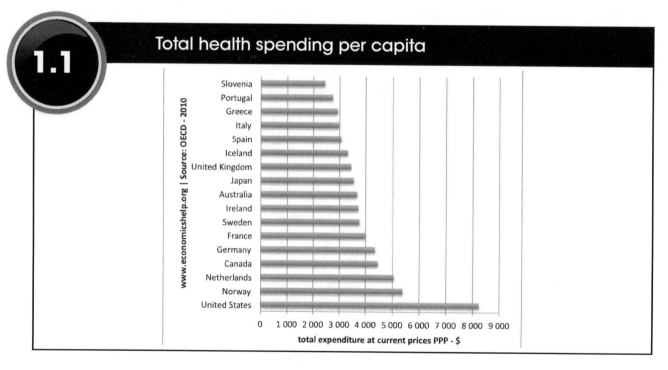

1.1 Total health spending per capita

National health spending is projected to increase as a share of GDP over the next decade.

Resources are limited, reimbursement is decreasing, and it has become imperative that nurse leaders control and/or manage costs on their units.

This big-picture perspective affects healthcare costs on a national scale. Each state has its own challenges and issues, and reimbursement by payer type may differ. Think about the baby boomers: By 2029, when the youngest boomer turns 65, there will be more than 71 million baby boomers. We can expect the related healthcare costs to continue to skyrocket.

The Financial Reimbursement Breakdown

Prior to 1983, hospitals were reimbursed for the services they provided by insurance companies or directly by the patient. This included such expenditures as room charges, nursing care, ancillary services, medications, procedures, linen, food, etc. Bills were sent to the insurance company or to patients. This system depended heavily on the nursing department and ancillary services. Cost containment was not an issue: The more hospitals charged, the more revenue they brought in. Management decisions such as the amount of staff or resources were essentially no-brainers because reimbursement was so healthy. Costs were shifted to insurance companies and patients, while hospitals enjoyed healthy financial statements.

However, after 1983, Medicare diagnosis-related groups (DRG) drastically changed hospital operations. DRGs categorize patient care by characteristics, such as diagnosis, treatment, age, and sex, to estimate patients' approximate length of stay (LOS) and use of hospital resources. DRGs are based on the prospective payment system (PPS), which determines the amount that hospitals can charge (hospitals cannot charge for all costs incurred for patient care).

Under PPS, hospitals could no longer charge for costs they incurred. Rather, their reimbursement relied on predetermined prices set by the DRG. Because of this shift in reimbursement practices, many hospitals began providing patients with the lowest level of care possible to control costs. With approximately 700 DRG categories, hospitals are paid a flat-rate reimbursement on the discharge diagnosis regardless of the patient's LOS, tests, procedures, or supplies used. As a financial manager, you must know how much it costs your hospital to care for patients per day because the reimbursement may not cover the cost of care. Also, depending on the percentage of Medicare patients admitted and cared for, the hospital's bottom line can be negatively affected.

Other payers followed suit, and in the mid to late 1980s, insurance companies also began paying hospitals differently. As mentioned before, insurance companies were billed for services rendered, for which they would pay the hospital. Today, these important third-party payers no longer reimburse hospitals for services rendered: Rather, they base reimbursement on negotiated rates, contracts, and outcomes. These payers often constitute the majority of revenue for hospitals. Some methods of reimbursement from insurers include reimbursing a percentage of the charges, or a "per diem rate." The per diem rate is a negotiated rate that the hospital receives for reimbursement regardless of the actual services rendered. A healthy payer mix composed of primarily third-party payers has a significant effect on organizations' financial health. Hospitals with a large percentage of Medicare patients need to make an extra effort to control costs; however, there are times when Medicare actually pays more than some of the hospital-negotiated contracts.

Another significant payer is Medicaid, the state health insurance program for the medically indigent. Under Medicaid, services paid vary from state to state. Reimbursement is often paid at a flat rate.

Changes with reimbursement and healthcare reform

Beginning in 2008, CMS announced that Medicare will stop paying for eight reasonably preventable hospital-acquired conditions. This ruling is primarily due to the increasing concentration by payers on quality, patient safety, and hospital performance. CMS has established eight conditions in which the presence of complications and comorbidities, should they occur during the hospital stay, will no longer lead to a higher DRG payment. By 2012, more were added. These "never events" for which there will be no reimbursement are:

- Foreign object retained after surgery
- Air embolism
- Blood incompatibility
- Stage III and IV pressure ulcers
- Falls and trauma
  - » Fractures
  - » Dislocations
  - » Intracranial injuries
  - » Crushing injuries
  - » Burns
  - » Other injuries

- Manifestations of poor glycemic control
  - » Diabetic ketoacidosis
  - » Nonketotic hyperosmolar coma
  - » Hypoglycemic coma
  - » Secondary diabetes with ketoacidosis
  - » Secondary diabetes with hyperosmolarity
- Catheter-associated urinary tract infection (UTI)
- Vascular catheter-associated infection
- Surgical site infection, mediastinitis, following coronary artery bypass graft (CABG)
- Surgical site infection following bariatric surgery for obesity
  - » Laparoscopic gastric bypass
  - » Gastroenterostomy
  - » Laparoscopic gastric restrictive surgery
- Surgical site infection following certain orthopedic procedures
  - » Spine
  - » Neck
  - » Shoulder
  - » Elbow
- Surgical site infection following cardiac implantable electronic device (CIED)
- Deep vein thrombosis (DVT)/pulmonary embolism (PE) following certain orthopedic procedures:
  - » Total knee replacement
  - » Hip replacement
- Iatrogenic pneumothorax with venous catheterization

Source: CMS; *http://www.cms.gov/Medicare/Medicare-Fee-for-Service-Payment/HospitalAcqCond/ Hospital-Acquired_Conditions.html.*

As a manager, it is important to continually educate and monitor staff to ensure competency in all areas of responsibility. As you can see from these changes, mistakes can be costly.

Managed care

With the passage of the Health Maintenance Organization Act of 1973, alternative prepaid health plans began cropping up around the nation. By the mid-1980s, "managed care" entered the health-care arena, and hospitals were forced to adapt to a new reimbursement method. Managed care refers to the entire spectrum of available alternatives to the traditional fee-for-service mechanism used for provider reimbursement. It is a system that manages or controls healthcare costs by carefully monitoring resource utilization and, therefore, shifting the financial risk to hospitals. In other words, managed care puts the burden of managing costs on hospitals by expecting them to control the use of resources in order for them to receive optimal reimbursement rather than having third-party payers, such as the patient or insurance company, pay for services rendered.

Remembering the various abbreviations for the following managed care plans can be confusing, as there are many. For instance, there are HMOs, IPAs, PPOs—and the list goes on.

HMO

The most common form of managed care is the health maintenance organization (HMO). There are two types of HMOs:

1. The group model, in which physicians are actually employed by the HMO
2. The individual practitioner association (IPA) model, in which physicians maintain a private practice while serving both HMO and non-HMO patients

With both models, a population of patients, or "members," is enrolled for a prepaid fee known as the capitation charge. HMOs focus on preventive care with the ultimate goal of keeping members healthy and out of the hospital. The fewer services members use, the more money the HMO gets to keep. For these programs, a low census is a good sign. In fact, many organizations with capitated contracts have outpatient clinics, and they put health and wellness programs in place to keep patients out of hospital beds and only admit patients when absolutely necessary. Hospitals are then left to figure out creative, innovative ways to provide quality patient care at the lowest cost possible.

IPA

In the independent practice association (IPA) model, a group of privately practicing physicians join together to form a coalition that offers managed health organizations a full spectrum of services. These physicians continue to treat patients with third-party payers while serving HMO members. This model is highly controversial, as it raises many ethical questions regarding issues such as the average length of time physicians spend with HMO patients vs. other patients and the number of diagnostic tests physicians request for their HMO patients. These questions arise because in this model, the more resources physicians use, the less they are paid.

PPO

The preferred provider organization (PPO) is a negotiated arrangement between providers and third-party payers. When a physician joins the organization, he or she agrees to abide by the rules and standards within the PPO's reimbursement structure.

The Bigger Picture

As a financial manager, you should always keep the big picture in mind. For instance, even though you do not have control over the payer mix admitted to your unit, you need to know your hospital's payer mix. The payer mix may differ dramatically depending on your facility's geographic location. For instance, a large urban teaching hospital will likely have more uninsured patients than a small, suburban community hospital. Each patient-care unit is its own business, and as the nurse manager, you are the chief operating officer of that unit. Knowing the payer mix makeup, or how your hospital is reimbursed, helps you understand why LOS is so important and how using fewer resources equates to increased profit for the hospital.

Understanding the Revenue Cycle Flow

As nurse manager, you must have a basic understanding of how revenue flows into and out of the hospital. Figure 1.2 shows a typical revenue cycle.

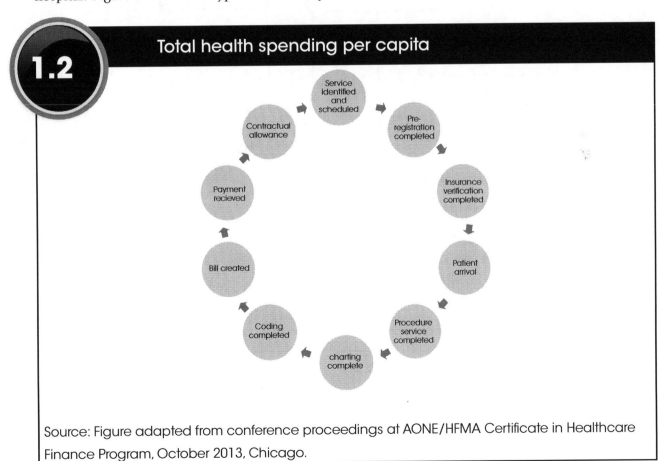

1.2

Total health spending per capita

Source: Figure adapted from conference proceedings at AONE/HFMA Certificate in Healthcare Finance Program, October 2013, Chicago.

Hospital hierarchy

In addition to understanding how revenue circulates throughout your hospital, it is also imperative that you know how professional power flows. Power flows are particularly important for nurse managers to know and understand because you deal with and present budgets to the financial experts within your organization. To get a better understanding of the typical financial hierarchy in hospitals, review Figure 1.3.

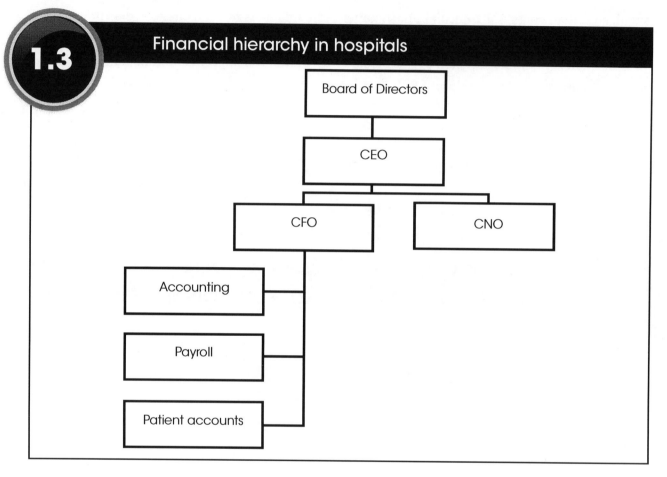

1.3 Financial hierarchy in hospitals

The governing board or board of directors is held accountable for the organization's financial performance and therefore has final approval of the budget. Board members are usually local business and community leaders who are not hospital employees. As the governing board, they empower the chief executive officer (CEO) to be responsible for the hospital's management, according to The Joint Commission's management standard. The CEO, in turn, empowers his or her administrative team to manage the organization's daily operations.

The chief financial officer (CFO) or vice president of finance heads the department, and he or she handles all of the hospital's financial operations. CFOs are employees of the hospital.

In the past, the CFO developed the budgets for each unit and presented them to the chief nursing officer (CNO). The CNO would then present that budget to his or her direct reports (i.e., nursing directors and managers). Today, most CNOs serve at the same level as CFOs and are expected to have the necessary financial and business skills to perform this expanded role. Likewise, nurse managers are now responsible for learning and understanding the tasks related to the financial aspects of their departments—including budget development—for which they are held accountable. In fact, The Joint Commission requires managers and staff to be involved in the budgeting process.

The finance department includes the accounting, payroll, and patient accounting divisions. The finance department manages the financial resources (i.e., cash, investments, and accounts receivable) of the hospital. This department or division is responsible for the following functions:

- Financial planning and auditing
- Accounting services
- Reimbursement and fiscal projects
- Data processing
- Patient financial services

Interdepartmental Communication

As nurse manager, hone your skills in communicating effectively with other departments. This is important because departments outside of nursing or outside of the cost center—the cost center being any department that accumulates costs—often affect your unit's business. For example, the nursing unit may be charged for biomedical services performed on unit equipment for preventive maintenance. Or, if nurses float to another unit, they may forget to charge their time to that unit. As nurse manager, you must know the cost and timing of such services so you can keep track of the money in your department's budget.

You must establish strong relationships not only with vendors and other clinical departments but also with the finance department. Engaging the finance department in the actual activities and services of your unit and maintaining healthy relationships with that team enables conversations to flow freely among units, allowing each department to express its needs. Waiting until your formal budget presentation is not a good time to negotiate what your unit needs.

Learning the Foreign Language of Finance

In nursing school, nurses are taught a vocabulary specific to the profession. To the untrained ear, this nursing language can seem confusing. It's the same with finance and accounting professionals: They use only their own terminology to communicate. Learn the language of finance to make your job easier and help you gain the respect of finance personnel.

Figure 1.4 lists some of the financial acronyms and abbreviations commonly used in hospitals. We will discuss each of these terms at length in Chapters 1 and 3.

1.4 Glossary of key acronyms and terms

ADC: average daily census

ALOS: average length of stay

Assets: liabilities + equity

CPUOS: cost per unit of service

FTE: full-time equivalent

Gross revenue: charges

HMO: health maintenance organization

HPPD: hours per patient day

Liabilities: financial obligations or debt

LOS: length of stay

Non-productive time: non patient care time (holiday, inservice, jury duty)

Patient day: an admitted patient in a hospital bed at midnight

PPO: preferred provider organization

Productive time: actual patient care time

Productivity: output/input

PTO: paid time off

ROI: return on investment

RVU: relative value unit

SWB: salary, wages, and benefits

UOS: unit of service

Volume: number of patients, tests, visits, procedures, etc.

UOS: A unit of service (UOS) is the specific item the organization produces and delivers to its customers. For instance, the UOS in nursing departments is typically an admitted patient who is in the hospital bed at midnight. In ancillary departments, such as respiratory therapy, laboratory, and radiology, UOSs may be the number of treatments, tests, or doses given to a patient in a given time period (most commonly at midnight). As nurse manager, you may be responsible for managing both inpatient and outpatient areas as well as supervising an ancillary service. Therefore, it's important that you know how UOSs are measured. In the nursing example, the admitted patient in a hospital bed at midnight (the UOS) is the measurement. In ancillary departments, each procedure, depending on its complexity, is assigned a relative value unit (RVU). For instance, with respiratory therapy, setting up oxygen may count as one RVU, whereas checking a ventilator may be allocated four RVUs.

ADC: The average daily census (ADC) is the number of admitted patients (inpatients) on any given day. However, depending on a hospital's operation, this may include observation patients. To determine the ADC, you divide the number of patient days in a given period by the number of days in that period. For example, in a nursing unit that is budgeted to use 7,500 UOSs per year, divide the number of UOSs by the number of days in a year (365) to find out the ADC. So, 7,500 / 365 = 20.55 average patients on the unit per day.

ALOS: The average length of stay (ALOS) is the average number of days patients spent in the hospital. Find this by dividing the number of patient days in a given period by the number of discharges in that period. For example, if your unit experienced 180 patient days and 50 discharges in one week, your ALOS would be 3.6 (180 / 50 = 3.6). Therefore, your patients stay in your unit for an average of 3.6 days.

CPUOS: The cost per UOS (CPUOS) is defined as the total cost of salaries divided by the units of service. You can use this financial measurement for any expense that occurs on the unit, but it is primarily used for salaries. To calculate salary CPUOS, take the total worked hours by staff and multiply it by the hourly rate. Then divide that amount by the UOS for that unit. For example, if the total salaries were $102,000 and the UOS were 660 for the month, then the total CPUOS would be $154.55 ($102,000 / 660 = $154.55) for worked hours. You can also calculate the total CPUOS by adding in the non-worked hours. The breakdown of these two categories will be explained in a later chapter.

FTE: A full-time equivalent (FTE) is the equivalent of one full-time employee working for one year. This is generally calculated as 40 hours per week for 52 weeks or as a total of 2,080 paid hours per year. This includes both productive and nonproductive (i.e., vacation, sick, holiday) time. For example, two employees working half-time for one year equal one FTE. To calculate FTE, multiply the length of the shifts by the number of days worked. Then divide the total by 40 hours, the number of hours worked by a full-time employee. For example, if a nurse works three eight-hour shifts per week, the FTE would be 0.6 (8 X 3 = 24 / 40 = 0.6). An FTE isn't a person; it is 40 hours per week, so 1.0 FTE can be composed of several people working during the week. More on this in Chapter 3.

Volume: This term refers to the number of patients admitted or in the bed at midnight, the number of treatments, tests, or procedures patients undergo, and the number of meals served, etc.

Productivity: Simply stated, productivity is output divided by input. Productivity rates measure the input required for a unit of output. When put into practice in hospitals, productivity is the number of staff who were used—either by hours or dollars—divided by the number of UOS used (i.e., midnight census on inpatient units). By comparing the actual staffing hours with the staffing hours required—while taking patient acuity levels into consideration—you can determine the standard productivity measure used in hospitals.

These terms and acronyms are some of the basics used in hospitals today. Incorporate them into your daily vocabulary. Understanding these terms—and how they fit into the big picture—will enable you to be more efficient and productive in your role.

Summary

The nurse manager role is critical to the success of a hospital or healthcare organization. As nurse leaders, you should be familiar with health policy and healthcare reform. Include your staff when discussing reimbursement changes, the cost of quality, and basic budgeting. Nursing can make a huge difference in the financial health of an organization by ensuring that high quality care is provided to our patients.

'Talking the talk' scenario

Review the following scenario, and think about the correct and incorrect ways to handle the situation:

New nurse manager Carey Carrington runs a busy telemetry unit. The unit is particularly difficult to manage because it has 85 staff members and an ADC of 26 patients. Patients are constantly transferring in and out of the unit.

Each week, Carey's productivity report reflects a large variance toward the beginning of the week, but her unit's midnight census has remained consistent. When reviewing the previous month's staffing reports and admission/discharge/transfer data, Carey found that an average of 20 new patients flowed through the unit during the same 12-hour period every Tuesday. She discovered that the patients were not captured in the midnight census.

Carey is scheduled to meet with her supervisor in the morning. What should she say?

Incorrect: "Tuesdays are really busy on the unit; we are always short-staffed and some of my nurses are threatening to quit. I need to hire another nurse. Can you please sign this hiring form so I can take it to HR and begin advertising?"

Correct: "After collecting data and observing the unit for the past 90 days, I have found that as a result of the cardiac catheterization lab scheduling, we take on an average of five extra cases each Tuesday. Along with the added cases, the intensive care unit census is running to capacity. Therefore, we have turned over an average of 20 patients every Tuesday for the past three months. And although our productivity reports show an ADC of 26, we are actually caring for 46 patients over the course of the day.

"I would like approval to increase staffing on Tuesdays, and I will modify the schedule accordingly. Currently, we are reducing staff on Fridays because of the lowered census, which will help maintain the overall budgeted HPPD. I will explain the variances each month on the variance report. I anticipate the overall CPUOS to remain the same."

Bonus tools

You will find a financial terminology cheat sheet and the top five survival skills every manager should know with the downloadable tools for this book. Please visit *www.hcpro.com/downloads/12427* to access the downloads.

Financial Management and Basic Cost Accounting

Learning Objectives

After reading this chapter, learners will be able to:

- Identify the components of a financial statement
- Explain the differences between a balance sheet, income statement, departmental operating report, and income and departmental expenditures

Financial Reports

Various financial reports or statements indicate an organization's financial health, and it is imperative that you are able to read, analyze, and understand them. The financials portray a picture of the health of the organization; remember that hospitals and healthcare systems are in the business of healthcare, whether for-profit or not-for-profit. As clinicians, we are responsible for the health of our patients. The chief financial officer (CFO) is responsible for the health of the organization. Nurse managers need to link the clinical agenda with the financial agenda.

Have no fear: Understanding the terminology and practices related to finance management and accounting is a skill that you will pick up through practice. This chapter will introduce you to the basic principles of accounting and show you how to read and recognize financial statements.

When reviewing the sample statements throughout this chapter, be aware that your organization's statements and line items (i.e., purchased services) may read differently. Find out exactly which services/fees fall under the line items in your organization's financial statements.

Hospital Accounting

Every hospital or healthcare organization has a formal accounting system to track its finances. Whether you work at a for- or not-for-profit organization, the accounting terms, functions, and rules are basically the same. These rules are known as generally accepted accounting principles (GAAP). GAAP were established by the Financial Accounting Standards Board (FASB)—an organization that determines the standards for financial accounting and reporting.

The following financial equation is widely practiced in business:

Assets = Liabilities + Owner's equity

Assets are any tangible or intangible resources or property owned by the organization.

Examples of assets include cash, buildings, equipment, and inventory. Remember, cash is the only thing that can buy anything, so it is important to have cash in the bank.

Liabilities are the financial obligations or debts owed to others by the organization.

Examples of liabilities include accounts payable, wages payable, and bonds payable. The largest liabilities are typically salaries.

Owner's equity, or net worth, refers to the assets an organization or its owners possess. The difference between assets and liabilities = net worth or owners' equity. This number should be a positive number!

Financial Statements

Balance sheet

The most significant financial statement in a hospital is the balance sheet. The balance sheet is a document that outlines the organization's assets, liabilities, and net worth at a particular point in time. Its contents change daily. It acts as a snapshot of the hospital's financial state, showing what the hospital owes and owns. It affects the organization's credit line, which affects its ability to build, borrow, or grow.

The creation of net worth for not-for-profit hospitals occurs when there is an excess of revenues over expenses. When the same happens in for-profit institutions, the excess is referred to as profit. The profit is then divided among the shareholders, and any leftover money is reinvested into the facility for such projects as adding services or constructing a new wing.

When looking at a balance sheet for the first time, it is easy to become frustrated and overwhelmed. Just remember that once you view a few of them, you will learn exactly what to look for, and it will be a piece of cake. To help you read and understand a balance sheet, we dissect the sample balance sheet in Figure 2.1.

2.1 Salary summary from sample cost center report	2015	2014
Current assets		
Cash and investments	$500,000	$750,000
Accounts receivable		
Patient revenues less:	$5,000,000	$3,400,000
Bad debts	300,000	150,000
Charitable allowances	50,000	50,000
Contractual allowances	450,000	375,000
Inventory	225,000	199,000
TOTAL CURRENT ASSETS	$4,925,000	$3,774,000

Fixed assets		
Land	$3,530,000	$3,530,000
Buildings (plant)	12,500,000	12,000,000
Equipment	4,500,000	3,500,000
Construction in progress	1,500,000	800,000
Total fixed assets	$22,030,000	19,830,000
Less: Depreciation	3,800,000	2,700,000
NET FIXED ASSETS	18,230,000	17,130,000
TOTAL ASSETS	$23,155,000	$20,904,000
Current liabilities		
Accounts payable	$2,500,000	$1,500,000
Accrued compensation and benefits	250,000	350,000
Accrued liabilities (interest, physician payments)	100,000	90,000
Current portion of long-term debt	100,000	50,000
TOTAL CURRENT LIABILITIES	$2,950,000	$1,990,000
Long-term liabilities		
Bonds payable	$15,000,000	$14,000,000
Mortgage payable	500,000	650,000

Tip

Sometimes the last group of 000s is dropped from numbers, meaning that all the numbers have been rounded to the nearest thousand dollars. This is done on balance sheets and income statements to conserve space and make the report easier to read.

First, it's important to know that items on the balance sheet are placed in order of liquidity, from the most liquid to the least liquid. This means those assets that can be turned into cash quickly, also known as liquid assets, are positioned at the top of the balance sheet to show financial stability.

Current assets

Let's review the first section, current assets (Figure 2.2), from the balance sheet.

2.2	Current assets		
		2015	**2014**
Current assets			
Cash and investments		$500,000	$750,000
Accounts receivable			
Patient revenues less:		$5,000,000	$3,400,000
Bad debts		300,000	150,000
Charitable allowances		50,000	50,000
Contractual allowances		450,000	375,000
Inventory		225,000	199,000
TOTAL CURRENT ASSETS		$4,925,000	$3,774,000

Cash is the most liquid asset and is always listed first. Cash constitutes all cash on hand/in checking or savings accounts. This also includes short-term certificates of deposit.

Marketable securities, which are short-term investments such as stocks and bonds, usually are listed next. If the intent of the organization is to sell these stocks or bonds within one year, they are listed under current assets. However, if the organization plans to hold onto them for more than a year, such investments are listed under the fixed assets section.

Accounts receivable (AR) refers to the assets that the patient or insurer is responsible for paying. Invoices are sent to patients or insurers charging them for services incurred, and payment is expected within 30 days. Therefore, on the balance sheet, AR represents the amount of money owed to the hospital. Finance departments often report their aging accounts to the chief executive officer. These aging accounts are often categorized by days, such as zero to 30, 30–45, 45–60, and over 60. By referring to the age of the account, the hospital can then determine when to write off these uncollected accounts as **bad debt**, meaning that the hospital will not recoup the money.

Patient revenues are all of the charges made to insurance companies and patients for outstanding payments for the time period covered on the report.

Charitable allowances are the amount of money the hospital budgets for free care. Most organizations provide a certain amount of free care to patients who will never be able to pay for services. These charges are eventually written off.

Although a hospital's goal is to collect all the monies owed to it, not all AR are collectable. The term **contractual allowances** refers to the difference between the amount the hospital bills Medicare, Medicaid, or other third-party payers and the amount the hospital receives from them. Because of contractual allowances and bad debt, hospitals never receive 100% of what they bill.

Inventory represents all of the on-hand stock/supplies that the organization owns to provide services in the future. Some examples of inventory include linens, medications, tubing, and intravenous (IV) kits. Items in the inventory category are considered current assets because, if necessary, they can easily be converted into cash.

Fixed assets

Fixed assets are long-term assets that include property, equipment, land, and buildings.

Let's review the second section, fixed assets (Figure 2.3), from the balance sheet.

2.3 Fixed assets	2015	2014
Fixed assets		
Land	$3,530,000	$3,530,000
Buildings, (plant)	12,500,000	12,000,000
Equipment	4,500,000	3,500,000
Construction in progress	1,500,000	800,000
Total fixed assets	$22,030,000	$19,830,000
Less: Depreciation	3,800,000	2,700,000
NET FIXED ASSETS	$18,230,000	$17,130,000

Land is property owned by the organization. It includes the land that the hospital and other medical office buildings (MOB) reside on as well as land obtained for future development or use.

Buildings include the hospital itself, MOBs, clinics, pharmacies, laboratories, and nursing homes owned by the organization.

Equipment is materials or devices used within the hospital or its other facilities. Examples of equipment include computer tomography scanners, magnetic resonance imaging machines, and surgical and cardiac catheterization laboratory equipment.

Construction in progress is exactly as it sounds. It includes all structural additions or renovations being made to buildings, wings, or units owned by the organization.

Depreciation refers to the loss of value property undergoes when it ages or becomes obsolete. In other words, when fixed assets lose their value, they lose their effectiveness for the organization. Therefore, it is important to take eventual depreciation into consideration when purchasing or appraising the value of a fixed asset. However, know that calculating depreciation is typically a task for the finance department.

Net fixed assets is determined by subtracting depreciation from the total fixed assets. Use the numbers for 2015 in Figure 2.3 to calculate the sample hospital's net fixed assets: ($22,030,000 – $3,800,000 = $18,230,000 net fixed assets).

Current liabilities

Toward the bottom of the balance sheet, you will find liabilities and owner's equity. Liabilities on the sheet are divided into current and long-term. Current liabilities are the organization's obligations or debts that it expects to pay off within one year. Long-term liabilities, or long-term debts, are paid after a one-year period.

Let's review the current liabilities section (Figure 2.4) from the balance sheet.

2.4 Current liabilities	2015	2014
Current liabilities		
Accounts payable	$2,500,000	$1,500,000
Accrued compensation and benefits	250,000	350,000
Accrued liabilities (interest, physician payments)	100,000	90,000
Current portion of long-term debt	100,000	50,000
TOTAL CURRENT LIABILITIES	$2,950,000	$1,990,000

Accounts payable refers to unpaid balances with suppliers (i.e., medical and nonmedical supplies bought from pharmaceutical companies with credit).

Accrued compensation and benefits, or accrued wages payable, are salaries and benefits to be paid to employees. These accrue during the pay period cycle.

Other current liabilities

Notes payable are another form of current liabilities. They are short-term promissory notes owed to the bank or lending agency that must be repaid within one year. Taxes payable are also current liabilities and are taxes owed to the state, federal, or local government. For for-profit organizations, this means paying real estate, sales, and income taxes. Not-for-profit organizations do not have to pay taxes and are thus tax exempt. However, they must still pay taxes on unemployment benefits and workers' compensation. Some balance sheets also have a line item called "deferred revenues." The term refers to payment the hospital has received from an outside agency or employer for services that the hospital has not yet provided. For example, the hospital is contracted to give out flu shots to an organization, but until the shots are administered, the revenue is a liability.

Long-term liabilities

Long-term liabilities are debts that the organization plans to pay off at least 12 months after the date on the balance sheet. In other words, they are debts that the organization plans to settle after the 12-month payoff period allotted for current liabilities. Examples of long-term care liabilities include bonds payable and mortgage costs.

Let's review the long-term liabilities section (Figure 2.5) from the balance sheet.

2.5 Long-term liabilities	2015	2014
Long-term liabilities		
Bonds payable	$15,000,000	$14,000,000
Mortgage payable	500,000	650,000
Net worth	$4,705,000	$4,255,000

Bonds payable are bonds that the organization issues and therefore must make scheduled payments toward, with interest that it pays to the bondholder for the use of the bondholder's money. Bonds are written promises made by organizations, or issuers, to investors stating that money borrowed will be paid back with interest on a chosen date. Typically, bonds are paid back in five or more years. Hospitals issue or "float" bonds for various reasons (e.g., for additional capital to construct a building).

Mortgage payable is the monthly mortgage(s) the organization must pay, with interest, for a time period greater than 12 months.

Net worth

Net worth is the value or worth of an organization after paying off all of its debts or liabilities. Remember: Assets − liabilities = net worth (owner's equity).

Depending whether the organization is for-profit or not-for-profit, names for the net worth line on the balance sheet may vary. For instance, when dealing with a for-profit organization, this line is usually called either net worth or fund balance. It may also be called owner's or shareholder's equity. On a not-for-profit's balance sheet, however, you will see it called fund balance.

The net worth line usually includes detailed information, which may include stockholder's equity and "retained earnings." Retained earnings are earnings that the organization sets aside for future construction or expansion projects. These earnings represent the profit that is not distributed to shareholders or owners in the form of a dividend.

Income statement

The income statement is the second major financial statement for the organization. Also referred to as the profit and loss or operating statements, income statements summarize organizational and departmental revenue and expense activities. Healthcare organizations have steered away from using the term "profit and loss," as it implies that they are for-profit and that isn't always the case. You are responsible for understanding the departmental income statement. However, as with everything in healthcare, it's important to look at the larger picture to help yourself understand the smaller one.

Let's begin our breakdown of an income statement by looking at Figure 2.6.

2.6	**Sample income statement**		
	(Profit and loss) ($000s omitted)	**2015**	**2014**
Gross patient revenues			
Routine services		$23,000	$21,500
Inpatient ancillary		22,000	18,500
Outpatient ancillary		11,000	6,000
Other revenue		$500	150
TOTAL GROSS REVENUE		$56,500	$46,150

Deductions from revenue		
Bad debt	3,000	2,500
Governmental allowances	12,500	8,500
Insurance contracts	5,000	3,100
Charitable allowances	500	1,000
TOTAL DEDUCTIONS	$21,000	$14,100
NET REVENUE FROM PATIENTS	$35,500	$32,050
Operating expenses		
Salaries	14,800	13,500
Benefits	2,400	2,200
Supplies	4,850	3,950
Medical fees	1,300	1,200
Purchased services	5,000	3,800
Maintenance	1,800	1,600
Professional liability	400	300
Other	800	400
Depreciation	1,900	1,700
TOTAL OPERATING EXPENSES	$34,650	$29,950
NET (Pre-tax) INCOME FROM OPERATIONS	$850	$2,100
PERCENT OF NET REVENUE (MARGIN)	2.4%	6.5%

The purpose of an income statement is to see how effectively money flows into and out of an organization by comparing its income and expenses for a particular month or year with the figures for the same time period one year prior.

Gross patient revenues

Following GAAP principles, revenues from patients—the largest revenue source—are listed first on the income statement. Expenses are listed later in the statement, as they will be subtracted from the revenues. Let's review Figure 2.7, which shows gross patient revenues from the sample income statement.

2.7 Gross patient revenues		
(Note: $000s omitted)	**2015**	**2014**
Gross patient revenues		
Routine services	$23,000	$21,500
Inpatient ancillary	22,000	18,500
Outpatient ancillary	11,000	6,000
Other revenue	500	150
TOTAL GROSS REVENUE	$56,500	$46,150

Gross patient revenue is all charges for services that the hospital provided. Typically, such revenue is broken down into the following categories:

- Routine services, which include room charges, medication, food, etc.
- Inpatient ancillary, which includes respiratory therapy treatments, x-rays, physical therapy, etc.
- Outpatient ancillary, which includes short-stay surgical patients, therapy, etc.
- Other revenue, which refers to sales from the gift shop, cafeteria, etc.

Deductions from revenue

Let's break down deductions from revenue, shown in Figure 2.8.

2.8 Deductions from revenue		
(Note: $000s omitted)	**2015**	**2014**
Deductions from revenue		
Bad debt	3,000	2,500
Governmental allowances	12,500	8,500
Insurance contracts	5,000	3,100
Charitable allowances	500	1,000
TOTAL DEDUCTIONS	$21,000	$14,100

Deduction from revenue is the amount subtracted from the actual charges. Typically, such deductions include the following categories:

- Bad debt, which includes charges that will not be paid by patients who were expected to pay

- Governmental allowances, which include the Medicare or Medicaid discounts from full charges

- Insurance contracts, which are contracts, such as with health maintenance organizations or other providers' discounts, that have been negotiated and agreed to by the hospital

- Charitable allowances, or free care, which include those charges for which the hospital won't be reimbursed by patients who were not expected to pay

Contractual allowances are another deduction from revenue category that you might find on an income statement. This category includes Medicare, Medicaid, and other third-party payer discounts and shows the deductions from revenue versus the gross revenue.

Net revenue from patients

Net revenue from patients is calculated by subtracting the total deductions from the total gross revenue. Use the amounts from 2015 to 2014 in the sample hospital's income statement in Figure 2.6 to calculate net revenue from patients ($56,500 – $21,000 = $35,500 net revenue from patients).

Typically, for every dollar billed in healthcare today, only 25–30 cents is received. This means that when we look at gross revenue, it accounts for what has been charged. Net revenue is what we actually receive, which is nowhere near what we charged.

Operating expenses

Operating expenses are all of the costs necessary for running an organization. Let's review Figure 2.9, which shows the operating expenses from the income statement.

2.9 Operating expenses		
(Note: $000s omitted)	**2015**	**2014**
Operating expenses		
Salaries and wages	14,800	13,500
Benefits	2,400	2,200
Supplies	4,850	3,950
Medical fees	1,300	1,200
Purchased services	5,000	3,800
Maintenance expenses	1,800	1,600
Professional liability	400	300
Other expenses	800	400

Depreciation	1,900	1,700
Financing costs	1,400	1,300
TOTAL OPERATING EXPENSES	$34,650	$29,950

Salaries and wages are the largest expense for a hospital. This expense can be broken down further into direct and indirect salaries. Indirect salaries are given to caregivers who do not work directly with patients, such as management, secretarial, and administration. Direct and indirect costs are discussed further in Chapter 3.

Benefits for employees are another operating expense. Some benefits include medical, dental, and vision insurance and holiday, vacation, and sick pay. These and other benefits usually amount to between 25%–50% of wages, depending on the organization and the region of the United States.

Supplies generally include medical items, such as 4x4s, sutures, and catheters as well as nonmedical supplies, such as fax printer paper, pens, pencils, forms, etc.

Medical fees are those paid to physicians by a hospital for the work they do within the organization—for example, the monthly stipend a physician is paid for acting as the medical director of a particular service.

Purchased services could include fees for traveling nurses, outside contract labor, or entire outsourced services, such as housekeeping or nutritional services. Purchased services are a line on the income statement with which you'll become familiar, because you may use this section to pay for some nursing salaries. Check with your finance department to clearly understand what is coded in purchased services.

Maintenance expenses are those related to the upkeep and ongoing preventive care of the organization and its equipment.

Professional liability refers to the liability insurance premiums that the hospital must pay to cover potential lawsuits.

Other expenses are those that do not fit into the above categories. They might include cab fare for indigent patients, flowers for a holiday party, and other such expenses.

Depreciation, as previously discussed, is the loss in value the organization anticipates for its buildings or equipment. Although it's good to understand depreciation, as nurse manager, you are not responsible for calculating it—the finance department is.

Financing costs refer to the expenses an organization pays toward money it has borrowed to replace or improve the hospital or its equipment.

Net income from operations (also referred to as "margin")

Net income from operations is calculated by subtracting the total operating expenses from the net revenues received from patients. Use the figures for 2015 on the sample statement to calculate the net income from operations in Figure 2.6 ($35,500 – $34,650 = $850 net income for operations).

The percent of net revenue, also known as the operating margin or bottom line, is determined by dividing the net income from operations by the net revenue from patients. Use the figures from 2015 to calculate the percent of net revenue ($850 ÷ $35,500 = 0.024, or 2.4%).

A healthy bottom line, also called the "margin," is above zero. The margin can be referred to in terms of dollars or percentage. If the margin is below that, it indicates that the hospital is losing money. Most hospitals like the margin to be 3%–8%. With healthcare reform, managing the margin is critical. No margin, no mission!

Departmental income statement

The departmental income statement goes by many aliases, including cost center report, profit and loss statement, and trend report. For the purposes of this book, the departmental income statement is referred to as the cost center report.

You should receive these reports monthly and for multiple cost centers. A cost center is a unit of the hospital that accumulates costs. Such departments have distinct budgets for revenue and expenses, as well as managers assigned to control them. Each department is identified and tracked through these designated numbers. Many times, units are split into two or more cost centers for more effective management. For example, in the obstetrics department, labor and delivery may have a single, separate cost center from post-partum and nursery, even though one manager is responsible for all three areas. Depending on the organization's size, cost centers may be rolled up into one report. Often, each division will produce reports for several cost centers.

The financial data on cost center reports are divided into department, division, or total hospital categories. Each manager receives his or her own cost center report, whereas directors receive reports containing information for all their cost centers. The hospital report lists all the cost centers. For health systems with numerous hospitals, regional and national reports may be compiled. As nurse manager, you will not receive all of these reports. However, if you are interested in seeing them, ask your supervisor or finance department for access to them.

The difference between the departmental cost center reports and income statements for the entire hospital is that department reports thoroughly break down revenue and expenses by units and cost centers to help managers keep a close eye on the money going into and out of their units.

From the cost center report, you can track the revenue that came into the unit and the unit's operating costs for a chosen month and compare them to those for the same month one year prior. Another benefit of the cost center report is the cost per unit of service (CPUOS) breakdown, which divides both salaries and hours by the total units of service (UOS) used during a specific time period. Negative variances are noted in parentheses. As with the organizational income statement, revenue is at the top followed by expenses and a breakdown of CPUOS and hours per patient day (HPPD).

Let's review the sample cost center report in Figure 2.10. This sample depicts a nursing unit (telemetry), for which the unit of service is a patient day. For ancillary departments, the UOS is the specific item that department produces and delivers.

Revenue

When analyzing the cost center report in Figure 2.10, look at the revenue section. You will notice that more charges were made during June ($1,400,000) than were allowed for in the budget ($1,040,000). Remember: The total revenue constitutes charges before contractual allowances are made. In a given hospital, this number may be either gross revenue or net revenue, depending on whether the contractual allowances have been deducted at the unit level.

Although some hospitals use a contractual allowances line on the departmental report to show net revenue, the sample cost center report in Figure 2.10 only shows gross revenue. As you can see, the majority of revenue for this cost center comes from inpatient services, or inpatient revenue, with a small amount ($500) coming from outpatient services, or outpatient revenue, collected at some point during the year.

2.10 Sample cost center report

Department: Telemetry Manager: Susie Smith
Cost center: 6150
Period ending: June 30, 2015

Current Month					Description	Year to date				
Actual	Budget	Variance	Var %	Prior year	Revenue	Actual	Budget	Variance	Var %	Prior year
1,400,000	1,040,000	360,000	35%	915,000	Inpatient revenue	15,253,126	12,062,013	3,191,113	26%	13,748,936
0	0	0	0	0	Outpatient revenue	0	0	0	100%	250
1,400,000	1,040,000	360,000	35%	915,000	Total revenue	15,253,126	12,062,013	3,191,113	26%	13,749,186
					Expenses					
222,156	191,952	(30, 204)	(16%)	198,554	Salaries and wages	2,469,073	2,229,607	(39,466)	(11%)	2,359,006
105,005	90,000	(15,005)	(17%)	101,775	Benefits	302,404	313,963	11,559	4%	307,449
85,000	60,000	(25,000)	(42%)	54,332	Professional fees	1,118,881	728,346	390,535	(54%)	663,951
150	200	50	25%	188	Purchased services	2,338	1,150	1,188	(103%)	1,872
13,222	12,654	(568)	(5%)	11,952	Supplies	155,409	162,654	(7,245)	45%	145,739
1,500	600	(900)	(250%)	720	Other	6,050	1,942	4,108	(212%)	2,378
8,263	8,152	(111)	(1%)	8,152	Depreciation	105,968	106,942	974	(.9%)	106,942
435,296	363,558	(71,738)	(20%)	388,761	Total expenses	4,160,123	3,544,604	615,519	(17%)	3,644,795
					Statistics					
625	605	20	3%	645	UOS	8,224	7,642	582	8%	7,888
8,362	7,528	(834)	(11%)	8,109	Productive hours	107,651	93,239	14,412	(15%)	95,386
998	1,012	14	1%	975	Nonprod.hours	10,992	11,377	(385)	3%	11,445
9,360	8,540	(820)	(10%)	9,084	Total paid hours	118,643	104,616	14,027	(13%)	110,398
13.38	12.44	0.94	(7%)	12.57	Productive hours/ UOS	13.08	12.20	0.88	(7%)	12.09
14.98	14.12	0.86	(6%)	14.08	Paid hours/ UOS	14.43	13.68	0.75	(5%)	13.99

Key:

Prod hours/UOS = Total productive hours divided by UOS

Paid hours/UOS = Total paid hours divided by UOS

Variance = Actual minus budget

Variance % = Variance divided by budget

Prior year = Last year, same month, actual

(+) = Favorable expense variance

(–) = Unfavorable expense variance

As nurse manager, you do not have control over inpatient revenue; therefore, focus on the expenses in the report. Additionally, those reports show gross revenue, not net revenue. In Chapter 3, we will further discuss what managers control in their budget. For now, let's focus on expenses.

Expenses

Expenses are an important section in the cost center report that you need to understand. This is because expenses are a large part of what you are responsible for, such as staff's salaries and wages, which constitute the largest expenses. Cost center reports typically are broken down into the following job categories:

- Registered nurse (RN)
- Licensed practical/vocational nurse (LPN/LVN)
- Clerical
- Physical therapist
- Respiratory therapist
- Technician
- Pharmacist
- Assistant
- Other

However, in Figure 2.10, salaries are lumped into one.

Tip

If your cost center report does not have staff's salaries and wages broken down by job type, ask your finance department to create a report that does.

According to the sample cost center report, actual salaries and wages were at $222,156, which is $30,204 over budget. That means that the unit ended up using more or more expensive staff than was budgeted for. You must explain this negative variance of $30,204 to the administrative department. There are tools and tips to help you analyze and communicate your budget with others in Chapter 4.

Benefits were also over budget in June. According to the sample report, benefits include vacation and sick time, holidays, and education, such as conferences staff attended or meetings that were held. It also includes paid days off or earned time off.

You must know exactly how your hospital defines "benefits" because the term is often broken down further into vacation, holiday, sick, workers' compensation, education, training, etc. Some hospitals might lump this all together. If that is the case, ask the finance department for source documents so you can complete your analysis.

You also may see the benefits item referred to as nonproductive on some cost center reports. Although you will have little to do with this item, keep track of the amount of vacation and sick time used. Sick leave also may include workers' compensation payments, so check with the finance department for a clear definition of what constitutes sick leave.

Tip

Keep an eye out for the things that negatively affect benefits' variance, such as extended sick leaves, long-term employees with high amounts of unused vacation time transferring to your cost center, and increases in mandatory education that were not budgeted for (i.e., new equipment, inservices, new regulations, etc.).

For many organizations, **professional fees** are those paid out by the organization to obtain staff. Professional fees include those for medical/physician costs, outside agency RNs or LPNs, and travel nurses brought in for high census days. Salaries of agency staff employed with the hospital are included in regular salaries. Sometimes expenses for outside temporary staff are found under the "purchased services" category. In the sample cost center report, all outside temporary staff are found under the professional fees category. In hospitals that use a high number of travel nurses, depending on the mix of travel nurses and regular staff, it is possible that a unit would come in under budget for regular salaries and over budget for purchased services.

Purchased services may include travelers, repairs, maintenance, catering, and any outside contracts (e.g., the copy machine) or other purchased services that may be allocated to your cost center. For example, if your organization uses an outside agency to provide housekeeping, this expense may be charged to each individual cost center.

Supplies consist of IV solutions, pharmaceuticals, cleaning supplies, medical supplies, sutures, scrubs, office supplies, and minor equipment (e.g., otoscopes, thermometers). As with the other categories, supplies can be broken down if you would like more detailed information. In fact, the report can go into such detail that, if requested, you could find out the exact number of IV tubings or O^2 tubings used on your unit.

Other expenses include items such as outside travel (e.g., sending nurses to outside conferences), dues and subscriptions (e.g., *Physicians' Desk Reference* and nursing journals), and rent/lease charges for equipment (e.g., IV pumps, telemetry/ventilators).

Depreciation, as you can imagine, is listed as an expense. If the unit has large equipment that will lose value, it is listed in this category.

Total expenses

All monthly expenses are added together to determine operating expenses. The total is then compared to the current month's budget and the total for the same month of the prior year.

Statistics

The statistics, broken down by UOS, typically follow expenses on the cost center report. The total UOS, such as patients who are admitted and are in a bed at midnight, are added for the month, and the total is listed.

Productive hours refer to the actual hours worked. As expected, the actual productive hours (8,362 hours) were 834 hours higher than were budgeted (7,528 hours) because the unit cared for more patients than planned. However, when divided by the UOS, you can see that the productive hours per UOS (13.38), or HPPD, were higher than budgeted. You must defend this variance to the members of the administrative department. However, you cannot do so by telling them that your hours and dollars are higher because of higher volume, as that argument would not match the figures. The increase in hours (834 hours) was not proportionate to the increase in UOS (20).

The cost center report is one of the most important reports, as it provides a detailed summary of all of the financial activity on the unit. Become familiar with this report. It is imperative to your success.

Bonus tools

You will find cheat sheets of key income statement terms and key balance sheet terms every manager should know with the downloadable tools for this book. Please visit *www.hcpro.com/downloads/12427* to access the downloads.

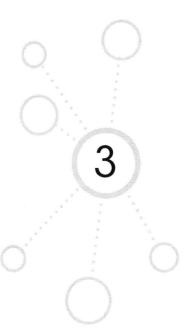

Building a Budget

Learning Objectives

After reading this chapter, learners will be able to:

- Describe the process of budgeting for staff, supplies, equipment, and capital expenditures
- Identify the process to construct a budget

The Budget Cycle

A budget is a financial plan that outlines the resources an entity foresees using for a particular time period. A budget quantifies activities into financial terms and represents management's expectations on comparing revenue and expenses. The master budget encompasses all the departmental budgets. Based on the organization's strategic goals and vision, the master budget is the actual statement of projected revenues and expenditures for the entire hospital.

Developing a budget is an ongoing process. See the budget cycle in Figure 3.1 to better understand the order and process of the budget cycle.

3.1 The budget cycle

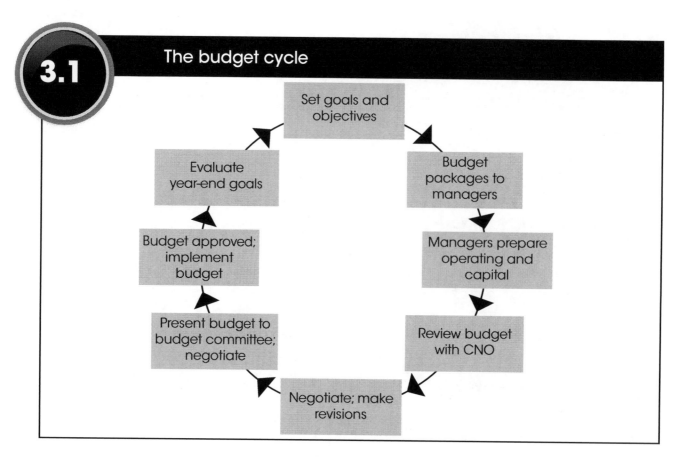

The budget cycle typically involves an environmental assessment that looks at trends in healthcare and in the hospital or healthcare organization, as well as among its competition. Once such assessments are completed, the hospital's goals and objectives are evaluated to determine whether any changes must be made. If changes must be made, the unit's goals are set based on the prior year's performance, trends in the marketplace, and assumptions about the future. The budget process should begin with a review of the organization's strategy and objectives, which forces the manager to establish unit goals.

The organization's operational objectives are developed and approved by the administrative department. It is at this point that the formal budget packages—including instructions, projected units of service (UOS), and revenue for the unit—are put together and distributed to department managers. Expect to receive such a package approximately four to six months before the budget is due.

Next, you will prepare your unit budget. At this point, negotiations between the nurse manager and the chief nursing officer (CNO), as well as any other departments, occur. Once the CNO approves your budget, you present it to the appropriate group(s), which usually consist of administration and the chief financial officer (CFO). The CFO will likely have questions that the manager needs to address. Following the meeting with administration and the CFO, you must make the necessary adjustments to your budget. If there is an opportunity to represent or appeal the budget, this is the time to do so. The budget is then approved, stamped, sealed, and ready to be implemented.

Finally, at the year's end, it is time to evaluate the annual budget. After doing so, you can determine what needs to be modified for next year's budget. Do this by tracking and trending activities and numbers throughout the year to develop a fair and reasonable budget for the following year. Collecting data by tracking and trending is the only way you will be able to negotiate for resources.

In many hospitals, the finance department and administration work together to develop a budget calendar. This calendar is distributed to all managers and helps keep everyone on the same page with their budgeting tasks for the upcoming year.

> ### Tip
> To review a sample budget calendar, look in the Chapter 3 folder with the book's downloadable tools.

At the end of the budget cycle, the hospital will create an operating budget that it must present to and get approved by the board of directors. For this presentation, all departmental budgets are rolled into one master budget. (The budget presentation is discussed in depth in Chapter 4.)

Controllable and Noncontrollable Expenses

You are responsible for managing the activities of your unit; therefore, you must know what you have control over. Typically, you control most of the activities on your unit that contribute to the budget. Such activities include staffing, skill mix, education, staff meetings, and orientation length. At the end of each month, you must explain to your supervisor any discrepancies in the numbers you budgeted. Internal accounting reports are usually given to managers. Such reports show the difference between the expected performance planned in the budget and the actual results. Managers have no power or authority to influence or change noncontrollable (sometimes called uncontrollable) expenses.

Your responsibilities are as follows:

1. Controllable expenses
   » Staffing
   » Orientation

» Skill mix

» Supplies

2. Noncontrollable expenses

» Patients' acuity levels and unit activity levels

» Types of benefits

» Regional overhead allocation

Types of Budgets

There are many types of budgets for which you may be responsible or to which you will make contributions.

Revenue budget

You may not be required to calculate revenue for your unit budget, especially if you are in an inpatient setting. You should understand the association of revenue with nursing care, but the finance department controls the charges (e.g., room charges) made to the patients on your unit. For managers who run a unit with multiple levels of care (e.g., medical-surgical and telemetry), the patient room charge is based on the level of care the patient receives on your unit. The level of care is typically based on staffing requirements or patient acuity levels. If a patient qualifies as high acuity, the hospital can charge more for his or her care, although Medicare will pay on the DRG, not acuity. Some of the indemnity plans will still cover these charges, but for the most part it really doesn't matter.

Outpatient areas typically have different reimbursement rates than inpatient areas. Therefore, managers who run outpatient areas, such as a clinic, emergency department, respiratory therapy, pharmacy, or other ancillary areas, may be required to calculate revenue for their budget.

Figure 3.2 depicts how the budgeted revenue is calculated for a unit with a UOS of 7,500 for the year.

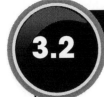

3.2

Sample budgeted revenue for med-surg/telemetry unit

(Unit with 26 bed capacity)
Budgeted UOS X room charge = budgeted revenue

Level 1 patients (medical-surgical)	4,000 x $700 = $2,800,000
Level 2 patients (telemetry)	3,500 x $900 = $3,150,000
Total budgeted revenue	**$5,950,000**

53% of all patients projected for next year will be Level 1 medical-surgical
(4,000 ÷ 7,500 = 0.53 or 53%)
47% of all patients projected for next year will be Level 2 telemetry
(3,500 ÷ 7,500 = 0.47 or 47%)

These percentages are determined by using historical data, trends in the market, and other contributing factors, such as insurance contracts and physician practice patterns.

Expense budget

Managers are typically involved in developing two types of budgets: operating and capital. The operating budget entails the unit's day-to-day plan for revenue and expenses. Most nursing units generate expenses, which might include the following:

1. Personnel expenses

   » Wages

   » Salaries

   » Benefits

   » Overtime

   » Orientation

   » Education

2. Other expenses

   » Supplies (medical and nonmedical)

   » Minor equipment

   » Linen

   » Purchased services

   » Maintenance

» Food

» Interdepartmental transfers

As you can see, expenses are broken down into two components: personnel and other expenses. Revenue budgets, such as physical therapy or radiology departments, are broken into inpatient and outpatient revenue.

Personnel budget

The finance department or your supervisor will determine the projected budgeted revenue for your unit, and then expenses must be calculated. As mentioned earlier, the biggest expense in the nursing department—and the hospital—is staff salaries. In fact, salaries often account for up to 75% of department and hospital budgets. The personnel budget determines how much staff is needed to operate the unit 24 hours a day, 365 days a year. When building your budget, most of your time will be spent here.

Budgeted staff in nursing includes the following and may include additional staff at your facility:

- Nurse manager

- Assistant nurse manager

- Charge nurses

- Registered nurses (RN)

- Licensed practical nurses (LPN)

- Nursing assistants (NA)

- Monitor technicians

- Orderlies

- Clerical staff

Budgeted staff in ancillary areas includes some of the following and may include additional staff at your facility:

- Department manager

- Assistant managers (if applicable)

- Pharmacist

- Physical therapist

- Respiratory therapist

- Lead technicians

- Technicians

- Assistants

- Clerical staff

The personnel budget is typically a variable budget—the numbers rise and fall depending on the volume and complexity of patient cases. For example, with inpatient areas, salaries increase or decrease depending on the volume of patients on the unit. The opposite of the variable budget is the fixed budget, which remains constant. Some ancillary areas have fixed budgets, but others do not. A fixed budget means that the department has fixed staffing or does not flex staffing with volume fluctuations. Some organizations use flex budgets. Flex budgets are created using budgeted revenue and expenses. A flex budget is adjusted, or flexed, to the actual census (at midnight) or activities (in ancillary departments) during the pay period or end of the month. So if the census goes above the budgeted ADC, the salaries, wages, benefits, supplies, etc., will increase relative to the increased ADC. Conversely, if the ADC or volume goes down, the flex budget will flex those expenses down as well. Check with your supervisor or finance department to clarify the type of budget you are responsible for and how you are expected to manage it.

In both inpatient and outpatient areas, other line items may be fixed, regardless of the volume. For example, if you allot $200 per month for minor equipment, this amount stays the same regardless of the volume of patient cases.

Budgeting Methods

Different organizations may have different budgeting practices. For instance, some hospitals use computerized programs to develop their budgets, while others calculate by hand. With some systems, nurse managers are handed a budget and asked to review, edit, and return it by a certain date; others are expected to perform zero-based budgeting (ZBB), which requires the manager to build a budget from scratch.

Zero-based budgeting

ZBB is the most effective and widely used method for budgeting. It consists of calculating projected costs by line item from the bottom up. In other words, rather than looking at the budget history, the new budget is built upon calculated assumptions. By using this method, you can analyze data and consider alternatives rather than relying solely on the previous year's numbers. Much of what is covered in the salary portion of expenses throughout this chapter resembles the ZBB method, but let's look at other models as well.

Flat percentage increase

The flat percentage increase method begins with a predetermined percentage, which is provided to you. This percentage is then added to the current actual number to determine the budget number. For example, assume that for eight months of salaries, year-to-date (YTD) expenses are $525,000. By figuring out the annualized number ($525,000 ÷ 8 months = $65,625 x 12 months = $787,500), you can then move to the next step. Multiply the annualized expense ($787,500) by the predetermined percentage (10%) to calculate next year's increase ($78,750). Add the increase to the annualized expense to reach the total expenses ($866,250) you can plan to pay for the next year.

Although this method is quick and easy, it does not take into consideration productivity, nor does it require analysis. It is important for you to look at the entire picture and learn from the previous year's experiences to produce a credible, realistic budget. Because of this, the ZBB method is most prominent in hospitals.

Budgeting software

Another way to calculate budgets is by using sophisticated computer software. Budgeting software has come a long way and is very user-friendly. Depending on the software, programs can be fairly expensive, but don't be discouraged if your hospital is not equipped with the software. The most important thing to remember is if your organization is willing to purchase such software, make sure your finance department approves it. In most cases, you will be provided with the software as those software purchasing decisions are made in the finance office.

Constructing Your Budget: Personnel Expenses

There are many steps related to determining personnel expenses for your budget. Much of the chapter discusses 13 steps you can take to calculate these expenses.

Step #1: Gathering data

To prepare your unit's annual budget, at a minimum, gather the following data regarding salary expenses:

1. Budgeted UOS or patient days

UOS projections may or may not include your input. Some hospitals provide managers the budgeted UOS and then assign them the responsibility of determining the needed personnel and other required resources based on those projections. Other hospitals negotiate with managers to determine UOS. Information used to determine UOS includes the previous year's actual UOS, projections for the upcoming year, and other factors, such as changes in the unit's physical layout, new programs or physicians arriving or leaving, and closing or opening of competing hospitals.

If you are told that your UOS is "flat," this means that next year your unit's UOS is expected to remain the same. If you do not agree with the projected or budgeted UOS for your new budget, present data to validate your assumptions (e.g., historical data or information regarding new patient classification types). Present these data early in the budgeting process.

2. Budgeted hours per patient day (HPPD)

To figure salary expenses, you must know the HPPD—or standard of productive, direct-care hours. HPPD is determined in a manner similar to UOS. To figure HPPD, hospitals will also look at benchmarks from national databases (e.g., those of HBSI International, Inc., or nursing associations) and compare the databases' data to the unit's operation figures. When comparing units, make sure that what constitutes the HPPD in other facilities is the same as in yours. For example, if your unit's HPPD includes orientation and education/training, don't compare your unit to one in a hospital that only looks at productive time. Think critically, and be willing to ask questions. Do not just accept these numbers from your finance department. In ancillary areas, the standard may be hours per visit, test, procedure, exam, or other.

For the purposes of calculating HPPD, assume that the nursing unit budgeted 67,500 hours the previous year. By dividing the total budgeted hours (67,500) by the UOS (7,500), the HPPD comes to 9.0 (67,500 ÷ 7,500 = 9.0). These hours are productive hours, not hours included with paid time off (PTO), jury duty, FMLA, etc.

3. Average and unit average hourly rates

Some organizations do not provide managers their unit HPPD but provide the total budgeted hours by job category, whereas others provide only a total salary dollar target and orders for the nurse manager not to be concerned with HPPD. When given the total budgeted hours by job category, determine the average hourly rate for the previous year. To do this, look at the total actual salary dollars for the previous year and divide that amount by the total hours worked. For example, if you paid $1,200,200 in productive salaries and used 65,700 total hours worked by staff, the average hourly rate for the previous year would be $18.27 ($1,200,000 ÷ 65,700 = $18.27).

Rather than breaking down the average hourly rates by job category, set a unit average hourly rate. Add together the hourly rates for each employee, and divide that total by the number of job categories. This number is determined by using the following equation:

(sum of hourly rates) ÷ number of job categories = unit average hourly rate

For example, if the average hourly rate for an RN is $35, for an LPN is $20, and for an NA is $12, then the unit average hourly rate equals $17.33 ([$25 + $18 + $9] ÷ 3 = $17.33). We will use this unit average hourly rate for future examples.

4. Skill mix

Another process you must become involved in is the skill mix breakdown. When determining this breakdown, take into consideration the type of nursing care model (i.e., primary nursing, total patient care, etc.), the hospital policy regarding use of LPNs and NAs, and patient acuity levels. In ancillary areas, the use of technicians or assistants would need to be considered. For the purposes of this book, use the following skill mix percentages: 75% RN, 10% LPN, and 15% NA.

Other considerations when calculating salary expenses

Productive and nonproductive hours: Salary expenses include productive hours (actual time worked or direct-care hours) and nonproductive (nonworked) hours. Nonproductive hours include orientation, education, vacation, sick time, holidays, etc. In preparing your budget, allocate required productive, or direct-care, hours. To determine productive hours, use the following equation: UOS x HPPD = total productive hours required.

For example, if the annual budgeted UOS is 7,500 and the budgeted HPPD is 9.0, then the total productive hours required is 67,500 (7,500 x 9.0 = 67,500).

Direct and indirect costs: Costs the unit incurs—and that you are responsible for—are called direct costs. Direct costs are those associated with the delivery of patient care. Some direct costs include salaries for RNs, LPNs, NAs, orderlies, and monitor technicians. Other examples of direct costs include supplies, administration fees, and electricity bills.

Indirect costs are those assigned to the unit from other areas. They are costs that are necessary for, but do not directly relate to, the delivery of patient care. For example, services from the bio-medical engineering department, or bio-med, fall under indirect costs. For instance, bio-med staff make routine inspections of nursing department equipment. Such maintenance costs are typically charged to the nursing department, because the service was for the unit where the patient received care; therefore, the bio-med department would not be charged.

Budget data

Review the budget data in Figure 3.3. It will be used throughout the chapter.

3.3 Sample budget data

Medical-surgical/telemetry (Unit has 26-bed capacity)

UOS: 7,500

HPPD: 9.0

Average hourly rate:	RN:	$25/hour
	LPN:	$18/hour
	NA:	$ 9/hour

| **Unit average hourly rate:** | $17.33 |

Skill mix:	RN:	75%
	LPN:	10%
	NA:	15%

Step #2: Calculating ADC

Next determine your unit's budgeted average daily census (ADC). ADC is important because it helps you explain variances and project staffing. It is needed also for subsequent calculations throughout this chapter. See the following exercise to get a better understanding of how ADC is calculated.

Exercise

What is your ADC?

UOS ÷ 365 or 7,500 ÷ 365 = 20.55

What is your budgeted occupancy rate?

ADC = 20.55 per day ÷ 26 beds x 100% = 79%

There are 67,500 productive hours budgeted for providing care to the ADC. The ADC represents 20.55 patients per day for 365 days.

Next, determine who will provide patient care and how. Remember that not all staff work full time; in fact, if you operate a 12-hour shift unit, each full-time employee will likely work 72 hours per pay period rather than the typical 40 hours.

Step #3: Calculating FTEs

Full-time equivalents (FTE) often suffer from mistaken identity. For instance, FTEs are thought to be people or jobs. In fact, FTEs are positions or hours worked. For example, two part-time RNs working half time will equate to one FTE, as their hours worked constitute the same as one full-time employee. One FTE equals 40 hours per week multiplied by 52 weeks, or 2,080 paid hours per year (some hospitals use 2,096 hours to calculate paid hours per year—check with your finance department). Therefore, no matter how many part-time employees work, if their total hours worked equals 80 hours for that two-week pay period, then they equate to one FTE. (See Figure 3.4.)

3.4 **FTE calculations**

Hours worked per two-week period ÷ 80 hours = FTE

RN	Hours worked per two-week (80 hours) period		FTE
Sally	80	(80 ÷ 80 = 1.0)	1.0
Joe	72	(72 ÷ 80 = 0.9)	0.9
Steve	64	(64 ÷ 80 = 0.8)	0.8
Nancy	40	(40 ÷ 80 = 0.5)	0.5
Sam	24	(24 ÷ 80 = 0.3)	0.3
Betty	8	(8 ÷ 80 = 0.1)	0.1
How many employees are there?	6		
How many FTEs are there? **3.6 FTEs**			

Note that with 12-hour shifts, staff typically work 36 hours per week for a total of 72 hours per pay period = 0.9 FTE. Although these employees are considered "full-time" and are entitled to full benefits, they still need to be replaced with a 0.1 FTE for budgeting purposes. This is a critical piece that is often missed in budgeting and staffing.

Now it's time to calculate the number of productive FTEs budgeted for this year. To do so, use the following equation: total productive hours ÷ number of paid hours within a year for an FTE = total productive FTEs (67,500 ÷ 2,080 = 32.45 FTEs). This number helps you calculate future data. Based on your HPPD and UOS, your unit is budgeted for 32.45 total productive FTEs.

Calculating FTEs by staff skill mix

According to Figure 3.3, the unit skill mix is 75% RN, 10% LVN, and 15% NA. Keeping that in mind, break down the FTEs further by their skill or job category. Do so by using the following equations:

75% (0.75) x 32.45 = 24.34 RN FTEs

10% (0.10) x 32.45 = 3.24 LPN FTEs

15% (0.15) x 32.45 = 4.87 NA FTEs

Total = 32.45 FTEs

Step #4: Determining average hourly rate

The average hourly rate becomes more important when determining salaries for the year. By using the average hourly rate, you avoid having to use each staff member's hourly rate. However, for a more accurate calculation of salary expenses for next year, use each staff member's salary. Because this process is time-consuming, we will use the average hourly rate for the RN, LPN, and NA job categories in this book.

The average hourly rate can be obtained from numerous sources. Look at your recent labor distribution report, staffing offices computer-generated reports, or payroll department report. No matter how you obtain the average hourly rate, make sure you do, because it's necessary for determining total direct salaries. Be sure to get the average hourly rate for each job category.

Figure 3.3 shows our assumptions for the sample medical-surgical/telemetry unit. Remember to factor in any projected merit increases/raises. To figure out the rate for each category, first determine the hours you will project for each productive category by using the following equations:

- RN total hours: 75% of 67,500 = 50,625 hours (0.75 x 67,500 = 50,625)
- LPN total hours: 10% of 67,500 = 6,750 hours (0.10 x 67,500 = 6,750)
- NA total hours: 15% of 67,500 = 10,125 hours (0.15 x 67,500 = 10,125)

Step #5: Calculating salary dollars by skill mix

In Figure 3.5, you will find the hours worked by each skill category (i.e., RN, LPN, and NA), the categories average hourly pay rate, and the total direct salaries you must account for in the department's budget.

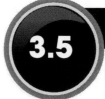

3.5 | Sample total salaries calculation

Hours x average hourly rate = Total direct salaries

RN: 50,625 x $25 =	$1,265,625
LPN: 6,750 x $18 =	$121,500
NA: 10,125 x $9 =	$91,125
Total direct salary dollars =	**$1,478,250**
When using the unit average hourly rate, use following calculation:	
67,500 x $17.33 = $1,169,775	$1,169,775

As you can see, by using the "average hourly rate" for each category in the equation, you are able to get a more accurate projection for salaries than when using the unit average hourly rate.

Step #6: Determining replacement needs

Figuring replacement hours by skill category

Using the information found in Figure 3.5, the nursing unit plans to spend approximately $1,478,250 for direct-care staff salaries for the year. However, when preparing your budget, remember that staff will take time off, and their replacements must be accounted for. To do so, first figure out the nonproductive hours, which will later be used to determine the cost of the replacement. The industry average for the percentage of nonproductive hours making up the total paid hours is 15%–20%. That means that 15%–20% of the money paid toward staff salaries is for nonproductive time (i.e., orientation, education, vacation, sick time, and holidays). This percentage varies depending on several factors such as the number of paid holidays the organization offers its employees as a benefit and orientation/education practices. The percentage of nonproductive hours is necessary when figuring FTEs and calculating the cost of salaries for the budget.

When budgeting for replacements, use 18% as the average (18% is the midpoint between 15% and 20%, the industry average). This means that 18% of the time, the employee from this skill or job category will not be working. Therefore, replace 18% of that time and cost for each staff category. See Figure 3.6.

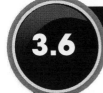

3.6

Calculating replacement FTEs

For varied skill mix:

How many replacement FTEs do you need?
18% (0.18) x RN FTEs (24.34) = 4.38—round to 4.4 FTEs
18% x LPN FTEs (3.24) = 0.583—round to 0.58 FTEs
18% x NA FTEs (4.87) = 0.876—round to 0.88 FTEs
Total additional FTEs needed for replacement: 5.86

For balanced skill mix:

If staff skill mix is balanced at 50%/50% (i.e., 50% are RNs and 50% are LPNs), another
way to calculate for replacement FTEs is by using the following equation:
Total FTEs x average replacement needed = Total additional FTEs needed for replacement
(32.45 x 0.18 = 5.84) Which is just about the same!

Now that you have figured out the additional FTEs needed for replacement staff, determine the new
totals for the FTEs needed for next year.

RN: 24.34 + 4.4 = 28.74

LPN: 3.24 + 0.58 = 3.82

NA: 4.87 + 0.88 = 5.75

Total projected FTEs: 38.31

Now it's time to determine the amount of additional salaries that must be accounted for
(nonproductive replacement) in the budget. See Figure 3.7.

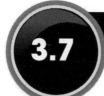

3.7 Determining nonproductive replacement

How much additional salary do you need to pay for staff's allotted time off?

Total direct salaries x average replacement needed = Nonproductive replacement
($1,478,250 (see Figure 3.5) x 0.18 = $266,085)

Total additional salaries needed for replacement (nonproductive replacement) of 5.86 FTEs: $266,085

Let's calculate the amount of productive hours per FTE. See Figure 3.8.

3.8 Calculating productive hours per FTE

**Adding cost of nonproductive replacement
and additional FTEs to productive**

Total direct salary dollars: $1,478,250	Total FTEs: 32.45 FTEs
Total nonproductive replacement: $266,085	Total nonproductive replacement: 5.86 FTEs
New total salaries: $1,744,335	Total FTEs 38.31 FTEs

Because we are using 18% as an average for replacement, we know that 82% (100% –18% = 82%) of the total paid 2,080 hours per FTE are productive. This is figured by multiplying the total paid hours per FTE by the percent of productive hours (2,080 x 82%). Therefore, there are 1,706 productive hours per FTE. The remainder of the 2,080 hours per employee is used for vacations, holidays, sick time, etc.

Step #7: Determining expenses for indirect positions

For this example, assume that the nurse manager and the monitor technician positions remain fixed.

Because the monitor technician is a 1.0 FTE on days, evenings, and nights and requires replacement, determine the total FTEs for this position by using the 18% replacement factor calculated earlier. For example, multiply the average replacement needed (18%) by monitor technician FTEs (3.0) to reach the nonproductive replacement (3.0 x 0.18 = 0.54). Then calculate the number of monitor technician FTEs by doing the following equation: 3.0 + 0.54 = 3.54 monitor technician FTEs. See Figure 3.9.

3.9 Sample position control

Position control for medical-surgical/telemetry unit

	Approved	Filled	Status
Fixed staff			
Nurse manager	1.0		
Monitor technician	3.54		
Total fixed staff	4.54		
Variable staff			
RN (includes charge nurse)	28.73 (75% of 38.31)		
LPN	3.83 (10% of 38.31)		
NA	5.75 (15% of 38.31)		
Total variable staff	38.31		
Total positions	42.85 FTEs		

To update the position control, list currently filled positions and their status. This allows you to see which positions are open. See Figure 3.10.

3.10 Updated position control for med-surg/telemetry unit

Position control for medical-surgical/telemetry unit

	Approved	Filled	Status
Fixed staff			
Nurse manager	1.0	1.0	0
Monitor technician	3.54	3.25	0.29
Total fixed staff	4.54	4.25	0.29
Variable staff			
RN (includes charge nurse)	28.73	26.75	-1.98
LPN	3.83	3.83	0
NA	5.75	6.0	+0.25
Total variable staff	38.31	36.58	1.73
Total positions:	**42.85**		
Total filled:		**40.83**	
Total open:			**2.02**

\+ FTEs are over the approved number

\- FTEs are under the approved number

You have calculated the direct salaries and replacements for the above salaries and FTEs. As you can see, other positions are considered indirect, as they do not provide hands-on patient care and are not part of the daily staffing hours. In this example, the nurse manager and monitor technician are considered indirect.

When adding the nurse manager and monitor technician's salaries, assume that the nurse manager earns $75,000 per year and the technician makes $10 per hour. To figure out how much of the budget can be spent on the monitor technician's position, multiply the approved FTE (3.54) by the pay rate of the position. Then multiply that total by the number of hours per year (3.54 x $10 x 2,080 = $73,632). Because the nurse manager is an FTE of 1.0 and is a salaried (or exempt) staff member, you do not have to multiply the salary amount by 2,080. To determine the total amount of indirect salary expenses that must be added to the current salary subtotal, add the two numbers together ($75,000 + $73,632 = $148,632). See Figure 3.11.

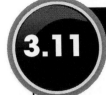

3.11

Determining total salaries	
Total direct salaries:	$1,478,250
Total nonproductive replacement:	$266,085
Subtotal salaries:	$1,744,335
Indirect staff salaries:	$148,632
Total salaries:	$1,892,967

Step #8: Calculating skill mix of staff per shift

Now that you have figured out staff salaries, determine the skill mix of staff per shift. Re-member that in some states, such as California, staffing ratios are mandated by law and dictate that nurses can only care for a specified number of patients at one time. There are currently other states in various phases of implementing staffing ratios, so keep your ears and eyes open for changing legislation. For the purposes of the following exercise, assume that no such ratios exist. To determine skill mix, consider factors such as your hospital's policy, the level of patient acuity, patient care history, and staff competency.

Your next action is to determine what percentage of nursing staff work days (7 a.m.–3 p.m.), evenings (3 p.m.–11 p.m.), and nights (11 p.m.–7 a.m.). Collaborate with staff when deciding the percentage of staff to work on each shift. For example, if the day shift is the busiest, consider putting most of your staff on the day shift. In units where activity does not change from shift to shift and shifts are generally eight hours long (e.g., critical care), the allocation may be 33%/33%/33%. This is because work is evenly distributed among all shifts. Keep in mind that, in most cases, most activities occur during day and evening shifts.

For an active, 12-hour shift unit (i.e., in an intensive care unit), it may be 50%/50%. As nurse manager, you control this number and can make changes based on the unit's activity. However, you should involve your staff when deciding the best way to distribute work over the 24-hour period. Because each organization is different, there are no set standards for staff distribution except in areas mandated by regulations. For this example, use the information given in Figure 3.12. Also for this example, assume that the following information is true:

- Budgeted ADC: 20.55

- HPPD: 9.0
- 75% of the staff are RNs
- 10% of the staff are LPNs
- 15% of the staff are NAs

Percentage of staff for each shift

Percentage of staff working days, evenings, and nights for medical-surgical/ telemetry unit

1. Total direct-care hours ÷ number of days in a year = total hours of care per day
   67,500 ÷ 365 = 184.93 hours of care per day
2. Total hours of care per day ÷ length of shift = shifts for 24-hour period
   184.93 ÷ 8 hours shifts = 23.12 shifts
3. Ask staff to make a list of tasks and activities that occur routinely on each shift. This list should include medications, procedures, physician visits, orders, baths, ambulation, etc. The number of tasks per shift will determine the percentage of staff needed on each shift. For example, there are a total of 100 tasks: 40 performed on the day shift, 35 on the evening shift, and 25 on the night shift.

Staff distribution by shift: 40% days, 35% evenings, 25% nights

The amount of hours of care per day (184.93 [67,500/365]) helps you calculate the number of staff members needed to care for the ADC of 20.55 patients for seven days a week, 365 days a year. Remember that FTEs are not shifts or people; they are positions or hours worked. To see what a 24-hour period would look like using the information calculated in Figure 3.12, review the chart in Figure 3.13. Using the following assumptions, you will be able to calculate how many shifts your department is allowed for a 24-hour period:

- Budgeted ADC: 20.55
- Total direct-care hours: 67,500
- Skill mix: 75% RN, 10% LPN, 15% NA
- Shift lengths: Eight hours
- Staff distribution by shift: 40% of X work days, 35% of X work evenings, 25% of X work nights

Use the following data to fill in the chart:

1. Total shifts for a 24-hour period

67,500 ÷ 365 days = 184.93 hours per day ÷ eight-hour shifts = 23.12 shifts for a 24-hour period

2. Shifts per staff category for a 24-hour period

- RN: 75% of 23.12 = 17.34 RN shifts for 24 hours

- LPN: 10% of 23.12 = 2.31 LPN shifts for 24 hours

- NA: 15% of 23.12 = 3.47 NA shifts for 24 hours

3. Number of staff needed to work shift

Days:

- 40% of the 17.34 RN shifts = 6.94

- 40% of the 2.31 LPN shifts = 0.92

- 40% of the 3.47 NA shifts = 1.39

Evenings:

- 35% of the 17.34 RN shifts = 6.07

- 35% of the 2.31 LPN shifts = 0.81

- 35% of the 3.47 NA shifts = 1.21

Nights:

- 25% of the 17.34 RN shifts = 4.34

- 25% of the 2.31 LPN shifts = 0.58

- 25% of the 3.47 NA shifts = 0.87

3.13 Calculating the number of shifts needed per 24 hours

Shift	Day (40%)	Evening (35%)	Night (25%)	Total
RN (75%) 17.34	6.94	6.07	4.34	
LPN (10%) 2.31	0.92	0.81	0.58	
NA (15%) 3.47	1.39	1.21	0.87	
Total	9.25	8.09	5.79	23.13

After plotting the calculated numbers, you will notice figures such as 0.92 and 1.39. These figures represent the number of shifts that must be filled and the amount of RNs, LPNs, or NAs needed to do so. Decide whether to round such figures up or down. For instance, for the day shift, you are allowed to fill the schedule with 6.94 RNs, 0.92 LPNs, or 1.39 NAs. You decide whether to schedule six RNs, one LPN, and two NAs or seven RNs, one LPN, and one NA. Whatever you decide, be sure to base your decision on important factors such as your state's staffing regulations, department activity, patient acuity, and nurse competency.

Figure 3.14 is a revised chart with rounded numbers.

3.14 Number of shifts allowed per 24 hours

Shift	Day (40%)	Evening (35%)	Night (25%)	Total
RN (75%) 17.34	7	6	4	
LPN (10%) 2.31	1	1	1	
NA (15%) 3.47	1	1	1	
Total	9	8	6	23
Total number of shifts allowed per 24 hours: 23.13 shifts				

Additional expenses

Additional salary expenses to add to the budget include shift differentials such as weekend bonuses, orientation, and benefits.

Step #9: Calculating differentials

Differentials are costs that the hospital pays to entice staff to work on the nonprime-time shifts such as evenings, nights, weekends, and holidays. Some hospitals will even pay a differential to nurses willing to fill in as charge nurse or to be a preceptor to a new grad or student. Differentials are used for those and other creative incentives to persuade staff to cover shifts they would not normally work. Every hospital pays some form of differential, so it's important that you add these costs into your budget. Earlier, we calculated the average hourly rate, which was calculated on base hourly pay only. When calculating the average hourly rate for your unit, remember to include differentials in your math.

For the sake of this example, assume the hospital pays the following differential for its medical-surgical/telemetry unit:

Staff	Shift	Differential
RN	3 p.m.–11 p.m.	$2.00
RN	11 p.m.–7 a.m.	$3.00
LPN	3 p.m.–11 p.m.	$1.50
LPN	11 p.m.–7 a.m.	$2.00
NA	3 p.m.–11 p.m.	$1.00
NA	11 p.m.–7 a.m.	$1.50

Remember that 40% of staff work the day shift, 35% work the evening shift, and 25% work the night shift. Use this information to calculate the additional salaries needed and add the sum to the salary subtotal. In other words, 40% of the staff will receive no differential because they are on the prime-time shift, 35% of the staff will receive the evening-shift differential, and 25% of the staff will receive the night-shift differential.

Determine the cost of such differentials by using the information we already have regarding skill mix and percentage of staff per shift. See Figures 3.15, 3.16, 3.17, and 3.18.

Calculating RN differential salary costs for evenings and nights

Total RN FTEs x percent working that shift = RN FTEs for the shift

Direct FTEs for RN: 75%

Total RN FTEs: 28.73

Work on evening shift: 35%   28.73 x 0.35 = 10.06 RN FTEs for the evening shift

Work on night shift: 25%   28.73 x 0.25 = 7.18 RN FTEs for the night shift

Average hourly rate (see Figure 3.3): $25/hour

RN FTE for the shift x differential expense x number of hours per year = differential salary expenses for RNs

Evening shift: 10.06 x $2 x 2,080 = $41,850

Night shift: 7.18 x $3 x 2,080 = $44,803

Calculating LPN differential salary costs for evenings and nights

Total LPN x percent working that shift = LPN FTEs for the shift

Direct FTEs for LPN: 10%

Total LPN FTEs: 3.82

Work on evening shift: 35%   3.82 x 0.35 = 1.34 LPN FTEs for the evening shift

Work on night shift: 25%   3.82 x 0.25 = 0.96 LPN FTEs for the night shift

Average hourly rate: $18/hour

LPN for the shift x differential expense x number of hours per year = differential salary expenses for LPNs

Evening shift: 1.34 x $1.50 x 2,080 = $4,181

Night shift: 0.96 x $2 x 2,080 = $3,994

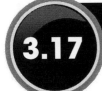

3.17   Calculating NA FTE differential salary costs for evenings and nights

Total NA FTEs x percent working that shift = NA FTEs for the shift

Direct FTEs for NA: 15%

Total NA FTEs: 5.75

Work on evening shift: 35%   5.75 x 0.35 = 2.01 NA FTEs for the evening shift

Work on night shift: 25%   5.75 x 0.25 = 1.43 NA FTEs for the night shift

Average hourly rate: $9/hour

NA FTE for the shift x differential expense x number of hours per year = differential salary expenses for NAs

Evening shift: 2.01 x $1 x 2,080 = $4,180

Night shift: 1.43 x $1.50 x 2,080 = $4,462

3.18   Total shift differentials

	Evening shift	Night shift	
RN	$41,850	$44,803	
LPN	4,181	3,994	
NA	4,180	4,462	
Total	50,211	53,259	$103,470

Step #10: Totaling salaries

Now that you've calculated shift differentials, re-tally the total for salaries and the budget. (See Step #6).

Total direct salaries: $1,478,250

Total nonproductive replacement: 266,085

Subtotal salaries: $1,744,335

Indirect staff salaries from above: 148,632

Total salaries: $1,892,967

Shift differentials: 103,470

New total: **$1,996,437**

If your hospital pays additional differentials to nurses filling in as charge nurses or serving as preceptors—above and beyond their normal salary—remember to add in the additional expenses to the final total. If the differential is $2.00 per hour and you use an average of 10 nurses per month on 8 hour shifts, the formula would be the following:

10 nurses x 8 hours x $2 = $8,320

Step #11: Figuring benefits

Benefits, or fringe benefits, are the last wages calculated and added to this section of expenses. Benefits are special perks given to those employed by the hospital. Such benefits may include medical, dental, vision, and life insurance. They also include pension and Social Security.

Today, depending where you live in the country, benefits can constitute up to 50% of salary expenses. Check with the finance department for your hospital's benefits percentage. For this example, use the benefits percentage of 30%. Add benefits to the total direct and indirect salary expense. To figure the amount of the budget spent on benefits, multiply the total salary expense by the percentage of benefits ($1,996,437 x 30% = $598,931).

Step #12: Calculating overtime

Pay close attention to incremental overtime. For instance, if staff routinely stay late to complete patient charts, talk, etc., their extra overtime minutes can add up. These minutes add up to hours, which adds to cost and FTEs.

If your hospital allows you to budget for overtime—some hospitals do not—review the previous year's data for your unit and calculate overtime at the hospital's overtime rate of pay. For example, if the overtime rate is time and a half and an RN makes $25/hour, the overtime rate of pay is $37.50/hour. To figure out how much overtime the RN would make, multiply the overtime rate of pay by the number of hours of overtime projected and the total added to the salaries. For example, assume that each RN works an average of 10 overtime hours per year. Use the following formula to calculate the cost of overtime:

Average overtime hours per year (10 hours) X overtime rate ($37.50) X the RN FTE (28.73) = Total cost of RN overtime (10 x $37.50 x 28.73 = $10,774).

Scheduled overtime is the overtime that is planned for in your budget. It can be the last four hours of a 12-hour shift or planned extra shifts. Some facilities are strict about overtime and only allow scheduled or 12-hour shift overtime to be budgeted with the understanding that the manager will control it on the unit. In such cases, overtime is not allowed unless it is an emergency. However, this practice is hospital-specific, so ask about your organization's policy. For this book, assume that no overtime has been budgeted for the coming year.

Step #13: Determining orientation and education/training costs

Orientation is the period of time set aside for new hires to learn unit policies and procedures and to become acclimated with its activities. Orientation consists of reading policies, observing experienced nurses, performing return demonstrations of tasks, caring for patients under supervision, and gaining understanding of unit practice standards.

When budgeting for orientation, either set money aside to pay for it or combine it with education. In some cases, orientation even may fall under productive hours. (It is important to understand where these orientation dollars are located so you can budget accordingly.) For instance, if you expect to absorb the orientation costs into productive HPPD, then factor this into your schedule. In other words, leave a buffer for those days when you have orientees on the unit. If you have a formalized nurse residency program, you will need to ascertain which cost center is paying the salaries during the residence, it may be a centralized area such as the education department. If not, you will need to add these hours and dollars to your budget.

Tip

To view six questions to keep in mind regarding orientation, look in the Chapter 3 folder with the book's downloadable tools.

Critical thinking

For this activity, assume that education, training, and orientation are separate from the HPPD and have a line item to themselves.

Facts:

- You will hire five new RNs and one LPN this year

- Each new RN and LPN requires six weeks of orientation on the day shift

- You will hire two new NAs this year

- Each new NA requires four weeks of orientation on the day shift

- Everyone on the staff is entitled to five paid education days per year

- All staff are paid to attend six two-hour-long staff meetings

- All staff are paid to attend four hours of cardiopulmonary resuscitation (CPR) training

- All RNs must take an eight-hour advanced cardiac life support (ACLS) course every two years

See Figures 3.19, 3.20, and 3.21.

3.19 Calculating orientation costs for new hires

Number of hires X length of orientation (in hours) X average hourly rate = total orientation costs

RN: 5 x 6 weeks (240 hours) x $25 = $ 30,000

LPN: 1 x 6 weeks (240 hours) x $18 = $4,320

NA: 2 x 4 weeks (160 hours) x $9 = $2,880

Total hours: 640 (total hours) ÷ by 2,080 = additional 0.3 FTE of staff for orientation. This number (0.3) must be added to the total budgeted FTEs.

3.20 Calculating education and training costs for new hires

FTE X paid education hours + (CPR training hours + staff meeting hours) = total education and training hours A

5 days = 40 hours, 4 hours + 12 hours = 16 hours, 40 + 12 = 56 hours

RN: 28.74 x 56 hours = 1,609 hours

Because the eight-hour ACLS is required every two years, you will budget 50% for the first year and 50% for the second. Therefore, only 50% of RNs will take the course this year.

50% of RNs x hours of ACLS training = total education and training hours B

50% of RNs (14.37) x 8 = 114.96, or 115 hours

(Total education and training hours A + total education and training hours B) x average hourly rate = total education and training costs

(1,609 + 115) x $25 = $43,100

FTE X paid education hours + (CPR training hours + staff meeting hours) x average hourly rate = total education and training hours

LPN: 3.82 x 56 hours x $18 = $3,851

NA: 5.75 x 56 hours x $9 = $2,898

3.21 Calculating total orientation and education/training costs for new hires

Total orientation costs + total education/training costs = total orientation and education/training costs

RN: $30,000 + 43,100 = $73,100

LPN: $4,320 + $3,851 = $8,171

NA: $2,880 + $2,898 = $5,778

Total orientation and education/training costs for RN + total for LPN + total for NA = total orientation and education/training costs

$73,100 + $8,171 + $5,778 = $87,049

You must add $87,049 orientation and education/training costs to the 2005 budget.

Now, total up the salaries for the budget:

Total direct salaries:	$1,478,250
Total nonproductive replacement:	266,085
Subtotal salaries:	$1,744,335
Indirect staff salaries from above:	148,632
Subtotal salaries:	$1,892,967
Shift differentials:	103,470
Benefits:	598,931
Subtotal salaries:	$2,595,368
Orientation:	87,049
Grand total salaries:	$2,682,417

Variable Costs Vs. Fixed Costs

For budgeting purposes, all costs are considered to be either fixed or variable. A variable cost is a cost or expense that is incurred as a direct result of volume (i.e., increased census or procedures or visits). A fixed cost is one the unit will experience regardless of the volume or activity (i.e., the electricity bill). The following are examples of both:

Variable costs	Fixed costs
Personnel	Electricity
Education	Depreciation
Food	Preventative maintenance

Supplies   Copy machine rental

Linen   Nurse manager salary

Variable costs are budgeted based on the UOS. That is because staffing, supplies, etc. use increases and decreases with patient census. Fixed costs, on the other hand, are often divided and budgeted as a flat monthly rate and do not change if the census does.

When budgeting for non-salary items such as supplies, the finance department should provide you with an "inflation factor." (If they do not, however, you must do the necessary research to obtain the number.) The inflation factor is a predetermined number accounting for price increases for the coming year. For the purposes of this chapter, assume that the inflation factor is 6%.

Annualizing Costs

One of the most common methods for annualizing costs is to look at the year-to-date (YTD) data on the most current departmental reports. "Annualizing" allows you to estimate the end-of-the-year, or YTD, numbers based on the unit's monthly history. Assuming that there is data for the past eight months (or however many months you have) to project expenses for the upcoming year, divide the YTD total—which is found on the departmental financial state-ment/cost-center report—by eight to get an average monthly expense. Then, multiply the sum by 12 months to reach an annualized number. For example, the YTD expenses for supplies is $35,000.

YTD expense ÷ number of months of data = average monthly expense X number of months in a year = annualized expense ($35,000 ÷ 8 = $4,375 x 12 = $52,500)

Although this method is not always exact, it does give you an estimate for average monthly expenses. After calculating the average for eight months of data, try to think of any significant expenses that may be incurred for the next four months that would be reflected in the average. If any, add them into the total. For example, if the average monthly expense is $4,375 and next month you expect to add a large volume of a new supply item to the supply cart, add this amount to the supply budget total. (See Figure 3.22.)

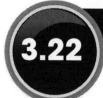

3.22 Methods for annualizing costs and planning expenses

Methods for annualizing costs and planning next year's expenses

Total fixed cost expenses YTD x 8 months x 12 months = Annualized figure

Fixed costs:

Bio-med costs for the last 8 months = $2,500.

($2,500 ÷ 8) x 12 months = $3,750 annualized figure

For next year's budget:

Annualized figure x inflation factor = Expenses for next year's budget

$3,750 x 6% (1.06) = $3,975 for next year's budget

Supplies

To determine supply expenses for the unit, review Figure 3.23.

3.23 Supply budgeting for a nursing unit

For the first eight months of this year, your unit consumed the following in supplies:

Medical = $23,967

$23,967 ÷ 8 x 12 = $35,951 x 1.06 = **$38,108 projected for next year**

Nonmedical = $12,006

$12,006 ÷ 8 x 12 = $18,009 x 1.06 = **$19,090 projected for next year**

Bonus tool

Test your critical thinking skills by figuring out what the projected expenses are for 2015. This exercise is in the Chapter 3 folder with the downloadable tools.

Plugging in your budget numbers

Now it's time to plot the above figures into your budget. See the example for the medical-surgical/ telemetry unit in Figure 3.24.

3.24 — 2015 budget for medical-surgical/telemetry unit

Medical-surgical/telemetry unit budget for 2015

Patient days	7,500
Revenue	5,950,000
Expenses	
Direct salaries	$1,478,250
Nonproductive salaries	266,085
Indirect salaries	148,632
Differentials/bonuses	103,470
Orientation/training	87,049
Overtime	0
Employee benefits	598,931
Total salaries	**$2,682,417**
Medical supplies	38,108
Nonmedical supplies	19,090
Minor equipment	1,800
Equipment rental	807
Maintenance	1,506
Bio-med	3,975
Linen	14,080
Nutritional support	20,948
Interdepartmental transfers	23,889
Other	1,109
Total expenses	**$2,807,729**

Capital Budgets

A capital budget is one that outlines projected purchase of large, fixed assets, like buildings, land, or equipment that depreciates, such as MRI or ultrasound machines. The capital budget is different from the operating budget (that you just built). What qualifies as a capital expense varies among organizations; however, generally, it is any piece of equipment that is worth more than $1,000 and has a lifespan of five years.

The capital budget is separate from the operating budget and requires all requests for capital equipment be approved by a budget committee. Granted requests must meet the goals and objectives of the hospital.

Most nurse managers are only responsible for their operating budget, while others may have a role in developing a capital budget. If you are responsible for developing a capital budget, you may have to fill out a form called the "capital budget acquisition form." Such forms are used when requesting funding for new equipment. They are used to make the case for purchasing new, large price-tag items and equipment. Check with your hospital to find out the policy.

Bonus tool

To view a sample capital budget acquisition form, look in the Chapter 3 folder with the downloadable tools.

Position Control

The position control or position budget (approved positions) discussed in step #7 is an important document and resource, second only to the budget itself. The position control identifies each job category, the number of budgeted FTEs, and whether projections are on target or there are vacant positions. The position control also indicates whether there are too many positions for a particular job category.

The position control comes in several varieties, and it was long thought that its only purpose was to serve as the "hiring plan" for the unit and for human resources (HR). However, when it is used as the translation of the budget into the defined "scheduling requirements" for the unit, it takes on greater importance in providing staffing for safe patient outcomes because there is consistent evidence for an association between the level of nursing staffing and patient outcomes.

Be sure to update the position control regularly as it changes each budget year or as your number of FTEs and skill mix change. In fact, update the position control each time a person is hired or when an employee resigns, transfers, or changes status.

Minimum, good, and best position control management

According to the Labor Management Institute, at a minimum, position control management addresses filled and open positions compared to hired and actual FTE positions.

Good position control addresses the minimum requirements as well as:

- Incorporates or references the budgeted FTEs by skill mix
- Positions by job codes or classes or skill mix (e.g., RN, LPN, NA) for direct care (defined as those that are part of the variable staffing plan providing hands-on care to the patient)
- Positions by job codes or classes or skill mix for indirect care (defined as those that are paid from the cost center but are not part of the variable staffing plan [also called fixed staff])

The "best" position control will include:

1. Job codes to track budgeted dollars for your FTE positions
2. Hire dates for the employees in the filled positions to track issues regarding seniority
3. Designation for full-time (FT) or part-time (PT) status as a check for your optimum or budgeted FT/PT rotation plan
4. Position control numbering schemas that allow for "loaning" filled positions to other units for some period (e.g., a diabetes educator that is hired to a unit for a diabetes education program that gets put on hold)
5. Position control reports that provide:
   - » Tracking by shift as a check against your budgeted "care distribution hours"
   - » Position tracking for weekday and weekend distribution to:
     - · Compare your budgeted positions to the schedule at posting to visually check that you have distributed your resources to the shifts to which they are budgeted
     - · Compare your budgeted positions to the schedule after the schedule is posted to visually establish where your resources ended up working, especially if you use self-scheduling in your unit (or selfish scheduling, depending on your unit-based guidelines and employee requests)
   - » Comparison of actual to budget paid FTEs with variance
   - » Comparison of actual worked FTEs to the target or variable staffing plan FTEs with variance
   - » Comparison of actual and budget workload for productivity reference (e.g., how busy the unit was for the period being evaluated)

Please refer to the position control example shown in Figure 3.25, which is the summary portion of the position control plan that demonstrates, integrates, and compares the unit's budget to the position control plan. It also contains the budgeted job codes, the position control numbers (e.g., 902.691.1201.1966.1) that incorporate the unit's cost center (902), the job code (e.g., 691), and the employee's hire date. You can also list the names of the employees occupying each slot.

3.25 Position control example

		700	1500	2300	Non-productive data		Perday	700	1500	2300
Unit Budget FTEs	43.7	14.6	14.6	14.6	Budget NP%	9.70%				
Position control FTEs	43.7	14.6	14.6	14.6	Budget NP hours	8,819.20	24	8	8	8
Hired FTEs	40.8				Budget NP FTEs	4.24				
Direct HPPD	19.5	6.5	6.5	6.5	Unit replacement NP FTE allocation	2.24	12.73			
Total HPPD	22.7	7.6	7.6	7.6	Resource Pool NP FTE Allocation	2	12			

Job Title	Job Code	Position Number	PC FTE	Hired FTE	Var. FTE	Filed By	Hire Date	Status	0700 Pos. Hours	1500 Pos. Hours	2300 Pos. Hours
RN Weekend Program											
	691	902.691.12011996.1	0.9	0.9	0	PT	12-01-1996	FT		32	40
	692	902.692.12121999.1	0.9	0.9	0	JC	12-12-1999	FT		32	40
		Filled RN Positions	31.8	31.8	0.05				9.35	12.15	10.3
		902.682.00000000.1	1	0	–1	Vacant					80
		902.682.00000000.2	1	0	–1	Vacant					80
		902.682.00000000.3	0.2	0	–0.2	Vacant					16
		Vacant RN Positions	2.2	0	2.3				0	0	2.2
		Total RNs=34.1	34.1	31.8	2.3				9.35	12.15	12.6
		Total RNs	34.1	31.8	2.3						
		Total Care Partners	3	2.5	0.6						
		Total Direct	37.1	34.2	2.9						
		Total Indirect	6.6	6.6	0						
		Total FTEs	43.7	40.8	2.9						

Overtime in excess of 5% is associated with adverse patient outcomes (medication errors and patient falls) based on research conducted by the Labor Management Institute, so position control reports that can tell us how efficiently and effectively we are scheduling and staffing our re-sources should help us to promote safe staffing for our patients. I recommend the Position Control Best

Practice Guidelines developed by the Labor Management Institute. See Figure 3.26 for the Labor Management Institute's criteria to help you evaluate your position control.

Figure 3.26

Labor Management Institute best practices position control

Criteria for evaluation of cost center position control:	Responses Yes	Responses No
1. Based on the budgeted FTEs		
2. Includes filled and unfilled (vacant FTEs)		
3. Includes category of staff (job codes/classes) or skill mix (for example, caregiver groups, such as direct (e.g., RN, LPN, NA, other) and indirect (e.g., unit manager, secretary)		
4. Includes date of hire for seniority tracking		
5. Includes positions for both full-time and part-time work agreements		
6. Allows positions to be distributed by shifts (days, pm, and nights)		
7. Allows positions to be distributed on weekends		
8. Compares budgeted positions to filled positions		
9. Compares actual hours worked by shift to the budgeted position		
10. Compares overtime by shift to the budgeted position		
11. Compares agency/traveler hours by shift to the budgeted positions		
12. Compares actual and budgted census or other workload for the reporting period		
13. Is manged by the unit manager		
14. Is shared by HR as the unit's hiring plan		
15. Is shared by finance for FTE management		
16. Is integrated to and updated automatically by HR, payroll, and workload information		
17. Provides reports that have been updated from integrated system data		

Once you determine the number of FTEs needed for the budget, develop a list of positions broken down by category. See Figure 3.9 for a sample position control for the medical-surgical/telemetry unit. Remember, the med-surg/telemetry unit has an ADC of 20.55 and 32.45 FTEs for direct caregivers. The position control includes fixed staff members who do not necessarily provide hands-on care but are in place regardless of the census. Such staff will not vary as the census fluctuates.

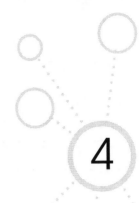

Budget Presentation and Unit Operations

Learning Objectives

After reading this chapter, learners will be able to:

- Describe breakeven analysis
- Define controllable costs
- Explain how to manage variances in their budget

Presentation Skills

Now that you have reviewed the concepts behind budgets and know how to build your own, it's time to learn the skills you need to successfully present your budget.

> **Tip**
>
> Practice your budget presentation with a peer, your director, or the chief nursing officer (CNO) before presenting it to the committee. This person can ask questions, which allows you to prepare answers before heading into the formal presentation. Doing a practice presentation also allows you to strengthen your presentation and public-speaking skills.

Presenting Your Budget to a Supervisor or Committee

First you must present the budget to your supervisor or the committee so the appropriate people can sign off on what you have proposed. Remember: No matter who signs off on the budget, you are held accountable for any discrepancies.

> **Tip**
>
> A budget is a budget. Never say "the budget is wrong." If there are discrepancies, indicate that you will provide a description of the issue or variance. Then develop an action plan to address the issue.

During the budget presentation, you will be asked whether the unit met its goals and objectives from the previous year. Be prepared to answer this question by explaining the current status of the goals and objectives as well as sharing your plans to modify the goals or develop new ones for the coming year.

Next, review the year-to-date (YTD) numbers from the current budget. The committee wants to know whether the YTD, or actual, numbers are above or below what you budgeted. Your job then is to explain any variances.

Monthly monitoring of the budget is crucial for being ready to answer the committee's or CFO's questions. By spotting trends and variances early, you can take advantage of opportunities or stop problems in their path. Either way, staying on top of your budget is the best preparation.

> **Tip**
>
> Bring data with you to your meeting. Trends that are depicted in a graph or a chart can be compelling. For example, if you can show that between 10 a.m. and 2 p.m. each day for six months your unit received 10 admissions, discharges, and transfers, this will provide you with data to build your case for more staff or HPPD.

After presenting your YTD numbers, discuss new programs or goals you either have established or wish to establish for next year. The bottom line: You need to be prepared for these discussions.

Variance Analysis

As mentioned earlier, variances are the difference between budgeted amounts and actual amounts. You must explain any variances on your monthly financial statements. Some organizations require managers to explain all variances, while others only require explanations for variances found in salaries, overtime, supplies, purchased services, or professional fees (i.e., any outside agency expense such as travel nurses or other agency staff, dues, subscriptions, outside education).

Do not waste time analyzing the areas over which you have little control, such as revenue or benefits. Instead, focus your energy on what you *do* control—staffing patterns, overtime, and the skill mix. In some hospitals, nurse managers must explain variances above 105% or below 95%, so know exactly what is expected of you before you begin your variance analysis. When doing your expense analysis, remember that variances over 100% are bad—this means you spent more than was budgeted. However, variances under 100% mean you spent less than was budgeted.

Remember to expect that when units of service (UOS) are on the high side, expenses in variable budgets will be higher as well. Therefore, when justifying your expenses over 100%, look at the UOS as well as other possible expenses directly affected by the UOS level. When dealing with revenue, however, it's good to come in over 100%, because it means that you were able to gain more revenue than was budgeted. Such gains often are due to an increase in the number of patients or complexity of those patients. However, as we learned in chapter 1, revenue = charges and the net revenue isn't reflected until after the contractual allowances are deducted. This does not occur at the unit level, so again, spending time analyzing your revenue, something you don't have control over, wouldn't be as productive as analyzing your expenses.

A lesson in variance analysis

To help you understand and analyze budget variances, let's review figures from the sample cost center report from Chapter 2 (Figure 2.10). The following excerpt (Figure 4.1) is taken from Figure 2.10 and includes analyses explaining each figure.

4.1 Salary summary from sample cost center report

	Actual	Budget	Variance	%	Prior year
Salaries	$222,156	$191,952	$30,204	(16%)	$198,544

Analysis: The salaries for this month were $30,204 over budget. This equates to a 16% negative variance (30,204 ÷ 191,952 = 0.16). You will need to explain this variance to your supervisor or the committee.

Another way to calculate percentage is: actual ÷ budget = variance
$222,156 ÷ $191,952 = 116%
This shows that you spent 16% more on salaries than the targeted 100%.

First, look at the UOS because, as noted earlier, nursing budgets are variable budgets, which means salary expenses increase and decrease depending on UOS. For example, if your unit cared for more patients than were budgeted, you can confidently predict that more money will have been spent on salaries than originally anticipated.

In ancillary areas, ascertain whether your budget is variable or fixed. In some instances, fixed areas are also required to "flex" staff depending on the hospital census. Check your hospital policy.

Look at Figure 4.2. Is the UOS higher or lower this month?

4.2 UOS summary from sample cost center report

	Actual	Budget	Variance	%	Prior year
UOS	625	605	20	3%	645

Analysis: The UOS was 20 more than budgeted for the month, meaning 20 extra patients received care. Does caring for 20 extra patients constitute spending $30,204 extra in salaries? Were the patients very sick? Was there a high acuity? Did staff work a lot of extra shifts, causing the unit to incur a large amount of overtime? As you can see, the UOS variance is only 3% over. This discovery makes it difficult to explain the 16% increase in salary expenses with only a 3% increase in UOS or patient case load (625 ÷ 605 = 103%).

At this point, take a look at the payroll report, an important source document. Typically, you will receive this report twice a month—assuming that there are two pay periods. While looking at the payroll report, seek out anything unusual (i.e., did another department code its time to your unit inadvertently?) If you cannot find any discrepancies, pull your admission/discharge/transfer list for the month. Most units keep this log themselves, but others must obtain it from the admissions or staffing offices. This list contains information such as the number of patients admitted to, transferred into and out of, or discharged from a unit for the entire month.

When reviewing the admission/discharge/transfer list, ask yourself whether the unit had an unexpected number of transfers in or out that were not reflected in the midnight census. Such patients were cared for by staff during the day but were transferred out by midnight, excluding them from the midnight census totals.

Figure 4.1 budgeted salaries of $191,952 divided by the monthly budget UOS of 605 (Figure 4.2) = Cost per unit of service (CPUOS) of $317. The actual salaries of $222,156 divided by the actual UOS of 625 = CPUOS is $367. This means that although you cared for more patients, the cost was higher than it should have been. This variance will need to be explained.

Now let's review supplies. See Figure 4.3.

4.3 Supplies summary from sample cost center report

	Actual	Budget	Variance	%	Prior year
Supplies	$13,222	$12,654	($568)	(4%)	$11,952

Analysis: Even though the unit was over by 20 patients this month, it still managed to go over budget by only $568, or 4%, for supplies ($13,222 ÷ $12,654 = 104%). This shows good supply management.

Because some hospitals have a "5% rule" that doesn't require managers to explain variance percentages of 5% or under, you may not have to explain that particular line item at all. Ask your supervisor or finance department about the organization's policy.

Let's look at purchased services. Analyze your budget's performance for these services by reviewing the summary in Figure 4.4.

4.4 Purchased services summary from sample cost center report

	Actual	Budget	Variance	%	Prior year
Purchased services	$85,000	$60,000	($25,000)	(42%)	$54,332

Analysis: As you can see, purchased services are a whopping 42% over budget at $25,000. If this is where outside agency costs are allocated, then the unit is significantly over budget. This is because salaries are already 16% over budget, and now purchased services (another line item that may be dedicated to staff salaries) are 42% over budget. If agency costs are included in purchased services, determine whether the hours worked match up with the dollars paid. In other words, sometimes when agencies are paid, the expense affects the budget in a different month than the one in which the hours were worked. The key is to research to find out. Because purchased services also can include housekeeping or other contracted services, it is important for you to break down this section by what is applicable to HPPD and salary costs. If this line item contains cost for only outside nursing staff, then it will be easier to figure out. If this is the case, combine the percent variance with the regular salary variance to obtain a true picture of the situation ($85,000 ÷ 60,000 = 142%).

To get to the bottom of this huge variance, look over the invoices that were paid for the month. Perhaps a large payment was made covering two months' fees for outside agency or travel nurses, or maybe someone prepaid a bill.

Locate the invoices and begin your analysis. Look for errors that may have caused your unit to be charged incorrectly. For instance, if the purchased services line item does not include nurse registry or nurse travelers, the unit may have been incorrectly charged for the indirect costs that are part of purchased services (e.g., housekeeping or nutritional services). It's important that you find out exactly which services are charged to this line item so you can monitor them accordingly.

4.5 'Other' summary from sample cost center report

	Actual	Budget	Variance	%	Prior year
Other	$1,500	$600	($900)	(250%)	$720

Analysis: The "other" line item covers expenses such as dues, subscriptions, and outside education. Find out exactly what is charged to this line item, because although the $1,500 actual is a relatively small number compared to the rest of the expenses, a 250% variance stands out greatly.

When building your budget, keep in mind that some costs do not change when volume fluctuates (e.g., subscriptions to monthly nursing journals or professional organization dues) and are divided over the 12-month period.

In this case, it looks as though a staff member attended a conference (perhaps it was prepaid) or dues were paid in a month you hadn't accounted for. Regardless, when you're presenting the budget, your explanation for this variance should echo your analysis of supply management. Also indicate that next month's charges for this line item will be minimal, if any at all.

Once you have reviewed, analyzed, and determined why the numbers were higher or lower than projected, communicate your findings to your boss. He or she may require that you develop and put in place a plan to bring the numbers back in order.

Once you have completed your variance analysis, document your findings to get your budget back on track. Many organizations use specific forms for documenting such information. View the sample variance report in Figure 4.6 below.

4.6 Sample variance report

Cost center: _____   Unit: _____

Month: _____   Manager: _____

Item	Actual	Budget	Variance	Explanation	Plan

Productivity Reporting

Productivity is how well you are able to control resources when delivering patient care. There are many formulas to determine productivity. However, one of the most popular for healthcare is:

output ÷ input = productivity

In the nursing department, productivity is measured by using the following formula:

number of hours required ÷ number of hours worked = productivity

For instance, say your weekly nursing productivity is 1,580 hours required, or the number of hours necessary to reach 100% productivity based on the budgeted average daily census (ADC) and hours per patient day (HPPD). Also, assume that the actual hours worked is 1,780. This shows that, for that week, the nursing department worked an additional 200 hours and was only at 89% productivity ($1,580 \div 1,780 = 0.89$ or 89%).

An example of daily productivity is when 152 hours are required and 160 hours are actually worked. The nursing department worked an additional eight hours, equaling 95% productivity.

Typically, charge or resource nurses are designated to complete the productivity form. This allows them to take part in managing the budget while creating ownership. Charge and resource nurses should be well-trained and have good leadership skills to fill this role. These individuals are also responsible for staffing and managing how such resources are used (e.g., the amount of staff used and the skill mix of staff).

After a 24-hour period, the completed productivity form as well as any written explanations regarding variances in staffing should be given to the nurse manager. The charge or resource nurse's documentation should also include any notes regarding activity, sick calls, floating (sending) of staff to or out of the unit, or other unforeseen events. Many of these reports are automated but should be reviewed for accuracy.

For the following examples, use an HPPD of 9.5 and a cost of per patient day (HPPD), or CPUOS, of $200 for the direct staff (i.e., registered nurses, licensed practical nurses, and nursing assistants). The nurse manager and monitor technician are indirect staff and are not included in the HPPD. Remember: productivity = output * input.

4.7 Sample productivity tool (HPPD)

Unit:

Date:

	7 a.m.–3 p.m.	3 p.m.–11 p.m.	11 p.m.–7 a.m.
Charge nurse			
RNs:			
LPNs:			
NAs:			
Inservice/orientation:			
Total:			
7 a.m.–3 p.m. total staff:			
3 p.m.–11 p.m. total staff:			
11 p.m.–7 a.m. total staff:			

24 hour total: _____ x 8 hours = _____ hours

Total hours: _____ ÷ midnight census _____ = _____ HPPD

Budgeted HPPD = 9.5

Comments:

Place in the nurse manager's inbox at the end of the night shift each morning.

As you can see in the completed productivity form in Figure 4.8, the charge nurses filled out the data, made some comments, and submitted to the nurse manager at the end of the 24-hour period. This allows the manager to have this data (busy evening shift, 5 transfers) to utilize on the variance report should he or she need it as the HPPD are higher than budgeted. A 24-hour period of time is only one snapshot in time, and he or she will need to keep an eye on the rest of the pay period to see if there are trends or issues.

4.8 Completed productivity tool (HPPD only)

Unit: Medical-surgical/telemetry

Date: 9/1/14

Nurse Manager: A. Jones (not included in direct hours)

	7 a.m.–3 p.m.	3 p.m.–11 p.m.	11 p.m.–7 a.m.
Charge nurse	N. Nelson RN	S. Smith RN	J. Jackson RN
RNs:	6	5	4
LPNs:	1	1	0
NAs:	2	1	1
Clerk: (indirect)	1	1	
Orientation: (direct)	1		
Total:	11	8	6
7 a.m–3 p.m. total staff:	11		
3 p.m.–11 p.m. total staff:	8		
11 p.m.–7 a.m. total staff:	6		

24 hour total: ____25____ x 8 hours = __200__ hours

Total hours: _____200_____ ÷ midnight census __19____ = _____10.53__ HPPD

Budgeted HPPD = __9.5__

Comments:

6 patients on telemetry with drips

5 transfers on day shift (not captured in MN census)

Busy 3 p.m.–11 p.m.

B. Brown IP, orientee 7 a.m.–3 p.m.

Place in the nurse manager's inbox at the end of the night shift each morning.

Patient Classification/Acuity Systems

Patient classification (or acuity) systems assist nurse managers in controlling costs and improving patient care while appropriately using financial resources. Within a nursing unit, patients are ranked at varying acuity levels depending on the complexity of care they require. Patient classi-fication systems are required by various regulatory bodies, including the Centers for Medicare & Medicaid Services' (CMS) *Conditions of Participation*, The Joint Commission, California's Title 22, and the American Nurses Association's Principles of Staffing. Check with your state to determine its specific requirements.

To measure the care needed for each patient, hospitals often assign a certain number of HPPD figures for each acuity level. Along with these acuity measurements come whole systems for classifying patients' complexity levels. Some of these systems are extremely intricate, while others are quite simple. Such systems may be computerized, off-the-shelf programs or created specifically for the needs of the hospital. Regardless of the sophistication of these programs, the more complex or ill the patient is, the more nursing resources they require.

For the medical-surgical/telemetry unit and HPPD of 9.5, assume that the noncomplex patients require fewer nursing care hours than more complex patients. As you may recall, when we built the budget, we calculated for a percentage of patients to be at the medical-surgical level and another percentage to be at the telemetry level in Figure 3.2. The reason for this is that we cannot determine the patient's acuity level until he or she is admitted and assessed. Looking back at the breakdown in Figure 3.2, 53% of our budgeted patients will be in the medical-surgical category (level 1), while the remaining 47% will be in the telemetry category (level 2).

Although the level 1 and 2 categories are used to guide you in assessing what types of patients your department will care for, you must use your unit-specific patient classification system to accurately assess the level of care required for each patient. In fact, when planning the budget, take patients' acuity levels into consideration so you can predict their care needs. For example, a patient awaiting discharge will require fewer hours of care than a patient who has multiple intravenous lines or limited mobility or who is dependent on complex procedures. Also use your patient classification/acuity system to monitor staffing and productivity. This is important because hospitals often staff by census, availability, or upon the requests of the charge nurse from the previous shift, which can put patient safety at risk. Another risky staffing practice is assigning a nurse—no matter what his or her competency level—to a certain area rather than basing workloads on patient acuity levels and staff competence.

In terms of discharging patients, check your hospital's policy on discharge times. If a patient is discharged, they should leave the unit soon after to open that bed for another patient. Often times, patients sit in their bed, waiting for a ride or for medications or supplies. This is costly, as staff is needed to care for them even though their acuity level is very low. In order to accommodate emergency department or direct admits, these patients need to be discharged in a timely manner.

Performing a Breakeven Analysis

Once you determine the budgeted ADC (see Step #2 in Chapter 3), make sure that maintaining this census is both profitable and safe. In Chapter 3, it was determined that the unit would run an ADC of 20.55. Now let's see whether this is a financially appropriate census. There are minimum staffing levels for each unit. These levels are based on the following:

- State laws that define ratios for the number of patients per nurse
- Hospital policies
- Break and lunch coverage (i.e., who watches patients when the nurse caring for them is on a break or away at lunch)
- Unit logistics (i.e., the ability to watch all patients, which may require additional staff)
- Transfer unit activity (e.g., if there is a low census on the unit but you anticipate many admissions from other units, you may need to staff two nurses to prepare for the incoming patients)

The breakeven analysis helps you determine whether it's financially feasible to keep the unit open. Consider both direct and indirect costs. That's because the bill for indirect costs such as electricity, copy machines, fax lines, and phones must still be paid even if the unit is at low census or closed. It's up to you to know at what point or dollar amount the hospital begins to lose money on direct and indirect costs. Ask your finance department about such figures, because you must also articulate them to your supervisor and the committee.

To determine the unit breakeven census point, determine the minimum staff necessary per shift (Strasen, 1987). As an example, use the information listed in Figure 4.9. For the example, assume that the hospital's policy is to staff monitor technicians 24 hours a day, seven days a week regardless of census. Also assume that the nurse manager is not "flexed," or taken off, the unit. In other words, he or she works on the unit 40 hours a week, and the hours are spread out over seven days. In instances in which the unit is closed for long periods, the manager's hours stay the same as he or she will likely be assigned to take on additional duties, such as managing other units.

4.9 Calculating breakeven

Medical-surgical/telemetry unit
Minimum hours ÷ HPPD = breakeven point

Shift	RNs	Monitor technicians	Hours
7 a.m.–3 p.m.	2	1	24
3 p.m.–11 p.m.	2	1	24
11 p.m.–7 p.m.	2	1	24
Nurse manager	(40 hours ÷ 7 days)		5.7
Total hours			77.7

Minimum hours ÷ HPPD = breakeven point

77.7 ÷ 9.5 = **8.17 patients**

The telemetry unit must maintain a minimum ADC of 8.17 patients to cover the direct costs of staffing for the unit. If the census drops below 8.17, the unit will incur higher costs than are allotted for the HPPD of 9.5. For instance, if only 7 patients are cared for, then the HPPD would be 11.1 (77.7 ÷ 7 = 11.1).

Cutting a Budget

There are times when you must reevaluate or cut your budget mid-year. Unforeseen circumstances, such as the loss of key insurance contracts, heightened competition, or low census, lead to this necessary reevaluation. In fact, if the census remains below budget for any length of time, the administrative team may ask all departments to cut costs, consolidate patients, and close units, or they may mandate an organizationwide cut. In such cases, hospital administration may begin enforcing a mandatory paid time off policy, or its members may try to set an example by taking days off without pay. Other measures to address unforeseen circumstances include a "no overtime" policy, a temporary cease in hiring, consolidating positions, or, in some instances, layoffs.

Other Controllable Costs

Poor performers, dissatisfied staff, and turnover

Cost containment is not just about salaries and supply expenses. Monitoring staff's performance is equally important. Because the cost of poor performance is difficult to quantify, it must be taken seriously and kept under control with good management and leadership. Negativity, such as poor performance, turnover, and an unsatisfactory unit environment, weighs heavily on the budget. Considering that the bulk of your budget is spent on personnel, it's imperative that you understand the effect that such problems can have.

Unhappy or inadequately trained nurses can result in increased turnover and cause costly errors. It's for these reasons that you must provide each staff member the opportunity to learn and grow within the organization. The more satisfied nurses are, the longer they will stay employed with your hospital.

Although many people think unsatisfactory salaries drive nurses out of hospitals, other factors—such as professional treatment and positive work environment—consistently rate higher for employee satisfaction. As a manager, you must maintain open communication, be available to staff, and listen to their concerns—these are the core managerial skills that aid in staff retention. Practice of such skills may seem a lot to ask from a busy manager who has to worry about the unit's financials. However, keep in mind that one nurse can cost up to $150,000 to replace, depending on the area. Can your budget afford that?

Another of your responsibilities is counseling, and sometimes terminating, poor performers. In essence, you are the chief retention officer on your unit. In this role, decide the best approach for handling problem employees. You may have to face difficult decisions, such as firing a problem employee or deciding to counsel him or her and taking the risk of losing five other employees by keeping the problem employee on. Think about these dilemmas and how they affect both the budget and productivity.

Above all, talk with your staff. By regularly communicating with staff, you're more likely to learn about problems, such as disruptive physicians, inappropriate staffing, lack of supplies, and other work environment dilemmas, before they become large issues. When you learn of such problems, you then have an obligation to resolve them. If you don't talk with staff or attempt to improve such problems, your nurses will leave.

Patient care and staff education

Another area that requires constant monitoring is the quality of patient care. The cost of poor care can be expensive—and deadly. Medication errors and pressure ulcers result in lengthened patient stays and increased costs. In Chapter 1, we discussed the CMS reimbursement guidelines for certain preventable conditions. Patients who fall, infections, medical errors, and wrong site surgery, to name a few, will not be reimbursed. Nursing can make a difference in these areas and lead the way with changing practice to avoid "never events." Mistakes can be extremely costly.

To ensure that staff members are properly trained and can give the highest-quality care possible to your patients, offer them regular training to keep them up to date on the latest care techniques. Remember to budget for the education hours offered on your unit.

Orientation

Orientation costs can be significant, so control them whenever possible. If a clinical nurse specialist/staff educator is not the person in charge of orientation, evaluate the average length of the program. For instance, evaluate the performance of new hires at 30 and 90 days, then decide whether they are competent to care for the patients on your unit. Managers often extend orientation time, thinking that the longer a nurse is trained, the better. This is not necessarily the case. Instead, use orientation as a probation period to weed out poor performers.

It's important that you budget adequate dollars for orientation, because no nurse should be pulled off orientation prematurely to fill a staffing hole. Although it does occur, this risky practice not only jeopardizes the safety of patients but also affects the new nurse, as he or she may not be prepared to provide care alone.

Bonus tools

For a list of six questions to keep in mind when budgeting for orientation, education, and training, look in the Chapter 4 folder with the book's downloadable tools.

Annual performance reviews

The annual performance review is an evaluation of the staff's performance for the entire year. Just as you must closely manage the budget to evaluate its performance, you also must monitor your staff. By watching staff perform their jobs daily and consistently communicating with them, you will use the annual performance reviews most effectively.

To make the most of performance reviews, allow ample time for discussion—after all, you are talking to a person about the job he or she does every day and your opinion of the quality of that work. This is a meaningful process to staff and often one of the few times they get your undivided attention.

When going over performance reviews with staff, ask them for feedback about your performance—ask them whether you meet their needs. Also, ask staff for at least one suggestion regarding performance improvement on the unit. By doing this, you give them a safe outlet for expressing any concerns they may have. Be sure to allow time to review last year's goals and, later, work on the new goals together.

From a financial perspective, annual performance reviews may lead to increased salaries, as many hospitals base staff raises on performance. Other organizations may base raises on years of service or the staff's level of clinical expertise. Either way, every hospital allots a certain amount each year for salary increases. Find out what salary percentages your hospital is offering its staff, as the amount may change from year to year.

Building a Business Case

Learning Objectives

After reading this chapter, learners will be able to:

- Identify the components of a business case

- Understand return on investment (ROI)

- Articulate why building a business case is important to secure the resources you need

Reevaluating Your Plan

Occasionally, after your budget has been implemented, circumstances arise that require you to reevaluate your unit's financial plan. Such circumstances may include the following:

- Sustained high census. For instance, say your budgeted average daily census is 20.55, but for the past 90 days, census has remained consistently at 26, requiring you to use travel nurses, overtime, and agency staff.

- Change in physician practices. For example, if a physician who frequents your unit acquires a new skill, his or her patients may require additional hours of care. Also, staff may require additional training to accommodate the needs of such patients.

- Offering additional services. Occasionally, your hospital may need to offer a new service, such as outpatient care, to stay competitive. Say a physician makes appointments with his patients two days after discharge for follow-up outpatient care. He is forced to use the clinic across the street because your hospital doesn't offer such services, even though your unit has unused space perfect for performing such procedures.

- Restructuring physical logistics. Changing of physical logistics, such as mid-year layout changes to accommodate another office, patient room, kitchen, or other renovations over $25,000, can alter your budget. (Ask your supervisor about the amount of money necessary for building a plan, but know that plans are usually for big-ticket items rather than smaller projects, such as moving a nursing workstation to a new location.)

- Need for a clinical educator (CE) or clinical nurse specialist (CNS) or clinical nurse leader (CNL). You may want to hire a CE, CNS, or CNL to work with new staff to increase competency, become more efficient, decrease costs, decrease falls, or other important initiatives. Such a need is unit-specific and must be well-justified.

- Need for an additional full-time equivalent (FTE). If there are significant changes in volume, admissions, acuity, or other factors, you may need another staff member. Although the "budget is the budget," you may need to make a case for additional FTE. If so, presenting the business case clearly and effectively is important.

Regardless of the circumstance, you must know how to request additional services, staff, or funds. In some organizations, the annual budgeting process also involves developing a comprehensive business plan for the next year or for a prescribed period (i.e., a three-year plan aligned with the hospital's strategic plan) (Waxman, 2012). In this chapter, we will discuss how to write a business case, propose a formal business case, and present it to administration in a confident and professional way.

Business Planning

A business case is a written document that summarizes a business opportunity. It outlines what the management team can expect to gain and the steps it must follow to take advantage of the opportunity (Timmons, 1994). Business cases are tools and thus must be comprehensive. They also call your target audience to action. In the business world, for example, such proposals or plans are often written by outside vendors to persuade a particular company to do business with the vendor.

You may have an idea or want to try something different for improving efficiency on your unit, and if the request is large enough, you might find yourself required to prepare and present a business case to your supervisor. The case to your supervisor may be brief, perhaps only one or two pages long. If approved, he or she may ask that you formally draft a business plan with the information you presented.

A good way to test the waters when seeking to make large changes within your unit or the organization is by using pilot testing. Consider presenting a business case for a pilot project instead of making large, unfounded requests. Pilot projects act as testing grounds for system or procedural changes. Such projects must have definite start and finish dates to allow evaluation at the end.

Following the project's evaluation—assuming that it was successful and that you plan to take it further—you must write a formal business plan.

Because the terms "business plan," "business case," and "proposal" are sometimes used interchangeably, it's important to find out what the process is called in your organization and how it works. For example, some hospitals have a formal process and proposal template for preparing a business plan. Throughout this chapter, we will review the basic concepts for writing a business plan. These concepts can be modified to best suit your facility's protocol.

You may be asked to write a business case, or you may write one on your own. Examples of when you would need to write one are as follows:

- Development of a new service
- Development of a program to increase revenue
- Development of a new program to operate more efficiently
- Development of a new program to increase quality
- Development of a specific business opportunity for the organization
- Large equipment purchase

Once you identify the need for a new service, program, or piece of equipment, write a professional business case to present to senior leadership. Regardless of whether it's required in your hospital, writing such plans or proposals is a good skill to have. Also, the plan or proposal will serve as an outline for your argument when you are requesting funding for unplanned expenses.

Components of a business case

There are various guidelines for business cases and plans; many are listed in steps, many by sections. Although each facility may list them in a different order, the following components are necessary to every business plan:

1. Executive summary

Every business case begins with a brief executive summary. This summary introduces the key components of a business case. It allows busy executives who review many business cases a day to quickly glance over the plan's initiative. The length of the executive summary varies greatly depending on what you present. If you are presenting a business case, it may be two paragraphs long. An executive summary for a business plan—which is a detailed plan—may be closer to two pages in length.

Use the executive summary to describe the project's importance, the problem or issue it addresses, and how it fulfills the hospital's or organization's overall goals. End this section by describing how your proposal will improve the bottom line, bring in revenue, increase productivity, or decrease costs. When writing this section, consider your audience, and write directly for them. Do they know about the current situation on the unit that leads you to seek change? If your audience knows nothing of the situation, first explain the problem, and then give any necessary additional information.

Typically, the executive summary is written after the business case has been written, but it is the first page of the document.

Tip

When writing the executive summary—or any presentation, for that matter—learn who your audience is before you begin. Be sure to mold the presentation to your audience's needs and desires. If you are speaking to the chief executive officer, make sure that your presentation solves a problem that directly affects the hospital's bottom line or addresses specific regulations such as those mandated by The Joint Commission or the state.

Other things to factor into your presentation are relativity and timing. In other words, if your hospital chose to close its obstetrics business, then writing a business plan for an obstetrics clinic would be a waste of everyone's time, and you'd seem uninformed about the hospital. Timing also is important. For example, if you are requesting funding, be sure that your request does not follow closely on the heels of layoffs or after the executives have just revealed less than satisfactory financial statements to staff.

2. Description of the present situation, identification of the problem, and summary of existing conditions

Your description of the present situation should be a main focus of the business plan. This, of course, is because it explains the immediate need for the project/product. Be brief and concise when explaining the existing conditions. Administrative team members sit through many presentations, and they will appreciate your thorough yet to-the-point explanation of the issue and your proposed solution.

The components of this section include the following:

- Explain your need for the request

- Define current state and why it is not working

- Identify the gap in what is needed and what currently exists

- Who are the stakeholders involved?

Review the following sample description and summary to get an understanding of how to present an issue in the business proposal:

Because of the increase of short-stay patients on the unit during the week, activity on the unit has increased, rendering the current staffing patterns inadequate for the growth in volume. Also, these high-acuity patients are not reflected in our midnight census. Therefore, our productivity appears low, yet we are not meeting our budget.

3. Description of the new program/proposed solution

Use this section of the business proposal to offer your solution for the problem you just presented. Describe the procedure or equipment that you're requesting, which staff it will help or affect, and any procedural or budgetary changes it will impact.

The components of the section include the following:

- What is your solution to the problem?

- What do you propose to close the identified gap?

- Is the proposal in line with the organization's goals and objectives? Tell the reader how your proposal aligns with these goals and objectives.

- Do new regulations impact the program or product you are describing?

- Is safety or compliance a compelling reason to bring this forward?

Review the following sample description:

Hiring an additional 1.0 FTE of an RN will enable the unit to care for these short-stay patients in a more cost-effective, timely manner. This RN will also serve as the liaison to the physicians, staff, patients, and family members. He or she will be the point person for orders and questions.

4. Presentation of options

In this section of the business proposal, review all possible options for handling the situation presented earlier. This section provides the opportunity for you to present your proposed solution and other options to consider. Starting with the status quo enables the reader to understand what the ramifications will be if nothing is done. Will the organization lose money? Will patient safety be impacted? By doing so, you allow those making the decision to weigh all of the possible outcomes and make an informed decision. Address the following three options when presenting this section:

Option #1: Keep the status quo and do nothing. When stating the first option, fully explain the ramifications of allowing the project/product to remain the same. For example, you might say to the committee:

If we do not take care of the problem now, overtime expenses will continue to rise. Therefore, until we develop a mechanism accounting for the increased activity, we will continue to incur overtime.

Option #2: The proposed solution. Use this option to address anticipated costs, and share with the decision-makers the results you expect to see. Be sure to tell the committee specifically, with set dates, when you expect to start working on the project or to purchase equipment. For instance, you might tell the committee your proposed solution is to:

Hire an additional 1.0 FTE RN by November 1, 2015, to act as cardiac admissions/transfer/discharge nurse and patient educator. The RN's responsibilities include overseeing the admission/transfer process, patient education as it relates to discharge instructions, and the discharge itself. Develop a new cost center for all revenues for short-stay patients and related staff and supplies expenses.

Option #3: Back-up plan. If you have a secondary solution or back-up plan you would like to introduce, now is the time to do so. Because it's your second proposed solution, fully explain why it's not your first option and why you feel your original solution is better. Do this by listing the pros and cons of each. For example, you might tell the committee that your secondary solution is to:

Designate exclusive space and staff to care for short-stay patients rather than absorbing them into the unit. This calls for a complete business plan with a cost/benefit analysis, which most likely would not be completed solely by the nurse manager, as it would include other stakeholders and involve further analysis.

5. Market analysis

If you are proposing a new program or service, this section is important. However, it may not be needed for a business case such as an additional FTE. Use this section to explain why external market forces will help lead to the program's success. For extensive business plans, this includes a SWOT (strengths, weaknesses, opportunities, and threats) analysis. A SWOT analysis is a good way to allow the reader to appreciate the time you took to think through all of the potential positives and negatives of your proposal. Also include in this section the data you gathered to back your claims. Such data could include your admission/discharge/transfer data, projected cardiac catheterizations volume for the next six months, physician practice patterns, and so on. As an example, you might present the following to the committee:

Over the past six months, admissions for short-stay patients have increased by 25%. The unit receives an average of five short-stay patient transfers or admissions per day, which was not anticipated during the budget process. These patients are discharged before midnight and are not counted in the midnight census. After surveying other area hospitals, we have identified the best practice. We found that most hospitals designate specific areas to care for these patients. Other hospitals also assign cost centers for revenue and expenses, which the current nurse manager must manage.

6. Implementation plan

Now it's time to explain how you or your staff will put the new program/product into practice. Introduce a communication plan, which is a written plan explaining the method you will use to communicate all related changes to the stakeholders. This is done via a formal memorandum, by verbally explaining the project during staff meetings, or by sending out weekly e-mail updates about the project's progress. For example, you might share the following implementation plan with the committee:

We will develop the job description and determine the salary structure, and Human Resources will then post the position internally. We will accept resumés for 72 hours after the posting. Following, the manager will interview candidates with charge nurses from each shift. The top two candidates will be selected to interview with the physicians, nurse manager, and clinical nurse specialist. We then will make an offer to the most qualified individual, and upon acceptance, we will set the start date according to the unit schedule. (If the person hired is an internal staff member, we will make every effort to replace his or her position immediately.)

We will hold a mandatory staff meeting explaining the new position and its associated roles and responsibilities. We will also revise staffing schedules to include the position. Working with the finance department, we will establish a cost center number and a name for the area (e.g., short-stay unit or 3 West, short-stay). By working with the admissions office, we will develop a communication plan to ensure that patients are coded appropriately.

7. Timeline and schedule for implementation

Develop and insert a clear, realistic timeline in this section. Remember to take into consideration budget cycle, pay periods, holiday time, etc., because they affect the amount of time people can afford to spend working on the project. Include a clear, realistic timeline. Include dates and milestones.

Components of the section should include:

- How will you put the program into practice?

- How will you communicate the plan?

- How will it be rolled out?

- Who needs to be involved?

- What (if any) additional resources do you need?

- Who is in charge of the implementation?

Bonus tool

To review a sample timelines, look in the Chapter 5 folder with the book's downloadable tools.

8. Evaluation plan

The committee or your supervisor will want to know how the program/product is working and when you will evaluate its progress. Perhaps you plan to use productivity data to track the success of the program/product. Employee, physician, and patient satisfaction surveys are also great ways to monitor and evaluate progress.

Components of this section should include:

- How will the program be evaluated?

- What data and metrics will you use?

- How will you measure success?

- What does success look like?

As the presenter, it's up to you to set the evaluation date. Will the evaluation program begin in 90 days, six months, etc.? Examples of both when and how the evaluation process will be handled might be described as follows:

The program will be evaluated at 90 days and again at six months. The following will be used:

- Productivity and overtime reports
- New cost center monthly financial report
- Patient, physician, charge nurse, and other staff satisfaction surveys
- Length of stay

9. Financials

This section identifies what you are asking for in terms of money/labor. For extensive projects or equipment, you may have to develop a timeline that shows upfront costs, monthly costs/ expenses, and when revenues will offset the expenses. It must also demonstrate when the project will become profitable or when the return on investment (ROI) is expected to occur. The ROI is an important part of the analysis, particularly for the finance committee or administration. They'll want see whether this project/product will pay for itself within six months, two years, etc. Prepare such statements for a three- to four-year time period or until breakeven occurs. Breakeven is when revenues and expenses are the same, or when the project/product pays for itself. The faster you can show the breakeven point, the more likely your idea will be approved.

Within this section, you are expected to quantify the amount of money/labor needed for the new procedure or equipment. For example, your cost/benefit analysis might read:

1.0 (FTE) x 2,080 (number of paid hours per year) x $30 (average pay rate for RNs) = $62,400 per year. The new position does not require replacement because it is a Monday–Friday position. However, there are costs related to benefits; benefits are at 30%. The total salary expense equals $81,120.

Overtime expenses for last month were $5,400. Much of this is directly attributed to the additional staff needed to care for the short-stay patients. After implementing the new RN position, we expect this amount to decrease by 75%, creating a $48,600 savings anticipated by the third month of the project. As noted earlier, short-stay patient revenue is not being allocated to the unit cost center. It is recommended that a separate cost center be developed to track both revenue and expenses. The overall impact of this would be an increase in FTEs. However, it would be designated to the appropriate cost center and justified by the revenue from more lucrative outpatient procedures.

The financial presentation is the final component of the business plan. This is where you outline the bottom line and tell your audience how much the proposed solution will cost. In fact, you will notice many executives like to page through to this section right away to view the bottom line numbers. Because it is of such great importance to your audience, it is imperative that you have a clear depiction of this bottom line and pay off, or ROI. ROI is what the hospital can expect to gain from funding the proposed program/product (in this case, for the new RN position).

Tip

When preparing your financial presentation, keep it to one page. Remember: Your audience includes executives who are busy and look at many reports each day. Keep it short and to the point: the bottom line.

An example of the financial presentation might go as follows:

1.0 FTE x 2,080 x $30 = $62,400 per year. The new position does not require replacement because it is a Monday–Friday position. However, there are costs related to benefits; benefits are at 30%. The total salary expense equals $81,120.

Currently, overtime expenses for last month were $5,400. Much of this is directly attributed to the additional staff needed to care for the short-stay patients. By implementing the new RN position, we expect this amount to decrease by 75%, creating a $48,600 savings. However, some incremental overtime will exist.

Revenue from short-stay patients is currently being allocated to surgical services and is difficult to quantify. After working with the accounts receivable department and analyzing the list of short-stay patients over the last 90 days, we determined that we are receiving approximately $1,100 per patient in reimbursement.

We anticipate that with an ADC of five patients x five days a week x 50 weeks

(no surgeries scheduled during holidays) = 1,250 patients per year. Anticipated revenue of $1,100 per patient x 1,250 patients = $1,375,000

Revenue:	*$1,375,000*
Less expenses:	*$81,120 (new position)*
	$2,500 (supplies)
Profit/net income:	*$1,291,380*

This is a high-level projection/budget. If the proposal is approved, a complete budget will be developed adding indirect costs.

Preparation Is Key

Preparation is the first step in writing a business plan. To properly prepare, you must talk to stakeholders and collect data. In this case, speak to the surgery manager, physicians, and accounting department staff or whoever is in charge of revenue allocation. Also, speak with the admissions office, because they will ensure that short-stay admissions are coded to the new cost center; the staffing office so they understand which staff belong on each unit now that you manage two cost centers; and your supervisor.

Collecting historical data for the defined time period is also crucial for getting your business proposal approved. For instance, use the productivity tool (Figure 4.7) in Chapter 4 to help build your case. Future projections are also necessary, as they allow decision-makers a clear view of the program/product's value in the grand scheme of the hospital's operation. Make appointments with the departments affected by the change (admitting or accounting, in our example) so you can collect your data and get their buy-in and support. Never submit a plan without first having the support of affected departments/physicians. Inform any department, in detail, that will be affected.

Conclusion

As mentioned earlier in the book, whether for-profit or not-for-profit, hospitals are businesses. And hospital managers are expected to have skills similar to those who work in other industries. Such skills include proposal writing, business planning, and finance and budgeting. Another skill that is critical—and perhaps most important—to your success as a manager is the ability to converse at a professional level about the issues on your unit. You must be able to think critically about such issues and present and discuss well-thought-out solutions.

Figure 5.1 is an example of a short, concise business plan following the steps indicated in Chapter 5. Depending on the proposal or project, some of the steps may be consolidated, others may be expanded. Use this sample as a guide.

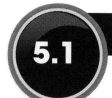

5.1 Sample business plan for a medical-surgical unit

Note: The following is a sample only, and most areas would need to be expanded for a real business plan.

Executive summary

As the hospital's patient population shifts more toward outpatient care, the number of short-stay patients is increasing. Short-stay patients are those that stay in the hospital for 23 hours or less and are then discharged to home. These patients are placed on the inpatient medical/surgical units for care and are not included in the midnight census. The staff salaries, necessary supplies, and room charge are charged to the surgical unit, yet the revenue from the short-stay patients is allocated to a different cost center.

After collecting data for a six-month period, it is evident that 5 West's productivity has been affected due to this unplanned volume of patients. We have an ongoing negative variance on our monthly cost center report and are not receiving credit for the increased number of patients in the midnight census. If we hire a 1.0 RN FTE to care for these short-stay patients and the unit manages both revenue and expense, we will decrease our overtime use significantly, which will yield cost savings.

Innovation in nursing at the microsystem level is one of the core values of the hospital and with this proposal, not only will we prove to be innovative, but the cost ($83,620)/ benefit ($1.2M) analysis estimates adding 1.0 RN position to be revenue positive, with return on investment being actualized soon after implementation.

Description of the present situation, identification of the problem, and summary of existing conditions

The medical/surgical unit is a 28-bed unit with an ADC of 2.5 and an occupancy rate of 85%. Because of an increase in the number of short-stay patients on the unit during the week, activity on the unit has increased, rendering the current staffing patterns inadequate for this growth in volume. Also, these high-acuity patients are not reflected in the midnight census. As the unit "absorbs" these patients to provide care, the staff salaries continue to be allocated to a different cost center, which increases our cost per patient day.

Presentation of options

Option #1

Do nothing and continue staffing as we have. If we do not address this problem soon, overtime expenses will continue to rise. Staff satisfaction has been affected, and we are at risk of losing key staff members. Therefore, until we develop a mechanism to account for the increased activity, we will continue to incur overtime and continue to use traveling nurses.

Option #2

Hire an additional 1.0 RN FTE by November 2015. This RN will act as an admission, discharge, transfer (ADT) nurse on the medical/surgical unit. The RN's responsibilities will include serving as a liaison to the physicians, staff, and family, overseeing the ADT process, providing patient education as it relates to discharge instructions, and facilitating the discharge itself.

Option #3

Designate exclusive space in the hospital to staff and care for the short-stay patients rather than "absorbing" them on the inpatient unit. This option would call for a complete business plan with a cost/benefit analysis, which most likely would not be completed solely by the nurse manager, as it would include other stakeholders such as engineering, finance, and other departments.

Develop a new cost center to address the revenue associated with short-stay patients and the expenses associated with nurses' salaries, supplies, linen, equipment, food, and other items. The current nurse manager of the medical/surgical unit will manage this cost center.

Market analysis

Over the past six months, admissions for short-stay patients have increased by 25%. The medical/surgical unit receives an average of five short-stay patient transfers or admissions per day, which was not anticipated during the budget process. These patients are discharged before midnight and are not counted in the midnight census. After surveying other area hospitals (total of four) and reviewing articles in journals regarding this topic (Smith and Jones, 2013), we have identified a best practice: We found that many hospitals designate specific areas in the hospital to care for these patients, particularly those hospitals with high volume.

Other hospitals also assign cost centers to monitor revenue and expenses, which the current nurse manager manages.

A SWOT analysis was performed, see (identify where to find the analysis. Note: a SWOT analysis has not been included in this book).

Implementation plan

Working with human resources (HR), we will develop a job description for the RN position and determine the salary structure. HR will post the new job internally prior to posting it in the local newspaper, job boards, social media, and schools of nursing. We will accept applications and resumes for 72 hours after the position has been posted.

Once qualified applicants have been identified, the nurse manager and the charge nurses from each shift will interview the candidates. The top two candidates will be selected to interview with two key physicians, the nurse manager, and the clinical nurse specialist on the unit. We will then select and make an offer to the most qualified individual, and upon acceptance, we will set the start date according to the unit schedule. (If the person hired is an internal staff member, we will make every effort to replace his or her position immediately, working closely with that nurse manager and HR.)

We will hold a mandatory staff meeting explaining the new position and its associated roles and responsibilities. We will also update the staffing schedules to reflect the new position. Working with the finance department, we will establish a cost center number and a name for the area (e.g., short-stay unit or 3 West, short-stay). By working with the admissions office, we will develop a communication plan to ensure that patients are coded appropriately. Additionally, we will develop a communication memo to all staff members regarding how to code their time on their time cards if they care for the short-stay patients.

Timeline and schedule for implementation
September 1–15: Develop job description
September 15–17: Post job internally followed by externally
September 17–25: Accept applications
September 25–October 14: Conduct interviews
October 14–16: Make offer
October 16–20: Meet with finance to secure cost center
October 20–22: Meet with admissions to review coding
November 2: Begin project with RN scheduled Monday–Friday

Evaluation of program

The program will be evaluated in 90 days and again at six months following the start of the program. Throughout the pilot period, we will conduct staff, physician and patient surveys. The following reports will be used in the evaluation after a baseline has been established:

- Productivity reports
- Overtime reports
- New cost center monthly financial reports
- Patient, physician, charge nurse, and staff satisfaction surveys
- Length of stay on medical surgical unit

Financials

1.0 FTE x 2,080 x $30 = $62,400 per year. The new position does not require replacement because it is a Monday–Friday position. However, there are costs related to benefits; benefits are at 30%. The total salary expense equals $81,120.

Currently, overtime expenses for last month were $5,400. Much of this is directly attributed to the additional staff needed to care for the short-stay patients. By implementing the new RN position, we expect this amount to decrease by 75%, creating a $48,600 savings. However, some incremental overtime will still exist. The overall effect of this change would be an increase in FTEs by 1.0. However, it would be designated to the appropriate cost center and justified by the revenue from more lucrative outpatient procedures.

Revenue from short-stay patients is currently being allocated to surgical services and is difficult to quantify. After working with the accounts receivable department and analyzing the list of short-stay patients over the past 90 days, we determined that we are receiving approximately $1,100 per patient in reimbursement.

We anticipate that with an ADC of five patients x five days per week x 50 weeks (no surgeries scheduled during holidays) = 1,250 patients per year. Anticipated revenue of $1,100 per patient x 1,250 patients = $1,375,000.

Revenue: $1,375,000

Less expenses: 81,120 (new position with benefits)

                        2,500 (supplies)

Profit/net income: $1,291,380

This is a high-level projection/budget. If the proposal is approved, a complete budget will be created that will include indirect costs.

**Note: Appendixes you may want to include: SWOT analysis, references, Excel spreadsheet for budget and other financials, job descriptions, GANTT chart, etc.